Amy Spangler's

BREASTFEEDING
A Parent's Guide

Amy Spangler, R.N., M.N., I.B.C.L.C.

Contributors
Doraine Bailey, M.A., *Breastfeeding and the Working Mother*
Rebecca F. Black, R.D./L.D., M.S., I.B.C.L.C., *Eating for Two*
Karen Kerkhoff Gromada, R.N., M.S.N., I.B.C.L.C., *Breastfeeding Multiples*
Winnie Kittiko, M.S.N., *Especially for Fathers*
Dennis L. Spangler, M.D., *Breastfeeding the Baby with a Family History of Allergic Disease*
Mary Rose Tully, M.P.H., I.B.C.L.C., *Breastfeeding the Premature Baby*

Illustrations and Production
Abby Drue, Inc.

Seventh Edition
Copyright ©2000 by Amy Kathryn Spangler, R.N., M.N., I.B.C.L.C. All rights reserved.
No part of this book may be reproduced without the written permission of the author.
Printed in the United States of America.

Previous editions copyrighted ©1985, 1987, 1988, 1990, 1992, 1995

ISBN 0-9627450-7-3

Library of Congress Catalog Card Number: 99-093780

To
my husband Dennis
my sons Matthew and Adam
my parents Phyllis and Elmer
my brother Mark
my friend Abby

Contents

Author's note:

Throughout this book, in an effort to keep the text clear and easy-to-read, the baby is referred to as *he* or *him* when a personal pronoun was necessary. The terms *milk* and *breastmilk*, when used, refer to human milk.

Foreword

Breastfeeding is the most precious gift a mother can give her baby. Breastfeeding has numerous advantages for both infant and mother. A woman preparing for childbirth needs to think about how she is going to feed her baby before the baby arrives. After a discussion with her obstetrician or midwife and, of course, with her partner, a woman needs some help and reinforcement about her decision as she continues to think about it. *Amy Spangler's BREASTFEEDING, A Parent's Guide* provides the information necessary to make a comfortable decision, thoroughly reviewing all the questions parents have. No woman is born knowing how to breastfeed, and it is not a reflex that develops; she must learn. Learning how to breastfeed is well-described in this parent's guide. It can be read and reread when breastfeeding is underway. Amy has made it clear and simple with her illustrations and instructions. It is pleasant reading.

As breastfeeding is initiated, questions may arise about the infant, the breasts, the milk, or the mother. The author has anticipated these questions and provides clear, concise answers. The discussion about less common problems that may occur is extremely valuable. It helps the reader determine what to watch for and when to call either the mother's or the infant's physician.

The highly publicized problems with breastfeeding are extremely rare and have been traced back in each case to the mother's lack of information about simple problems and the failure to ask for help from her health care provider. This book will be a reliable guide for parents in recognizing problems early and seeking help appropriately.

The author is an experienced nurse and mother who knows all phases of the childbirth process. Furthermore, Amy is an educator as well and knows how to share information in a clear, concise, complete manner. This parent's guide is an ideal source of information. Now in its seventh edition, it has been well-received by health care practitioners to supplement their patients' understanding of breastfeeding and provide an ongoing reference source about special situations. It is an excellent resource on both the art and the science of breastfeeding for parents.

Ruth A. Lawrence, M.D.
Professor of Pediatrics, Obstetrics, and Gynecology
University of Rochester School of Medicine and Dentistry
Rochester, New York

Preface

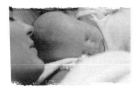

When I began teaching childbirth education classes almost 30 years ago, very few parents chose to breastfeed their babies. Fortunately, as knowledge of the benefits of breastfeeding has increased, so too has the choice to breastfeed.

I taught my first breastfeeding class in 1984. To encourage attendance, classes were taught in the evening and were provided free of charge. Knowing that many parents had never seen a baby breastfeed, breastfeeding mothers, fathers, and babies were included in each class. I wanted parents to see (and believe) that breastfeeding was easy, that breastfeeding was flexible, that breastfeeding was fun. I wanted parents to know that there were no rules or regulations.

In 1985, with the encouragement of the many parents I had taught, I wrote the first edition of *BREASTFEEDING, A Parent's Guide*. I understood that parents wanted a book that was clear, concise, and easy to read, not a dictionary, not an encyclopedia, not a medical textbook, but a simple yet complete guide to breastfeeding.

With the completion of the seventh edition, I marvel at how much I have learned since I wrote the first edition. While the art of breastfeeding has endured over centuries, knowledge of the science of breastfeeding has increased markedly in recent years. Today, parents choosing to breastfeed face unique challenges and seek realistic solutions. *BREASTFEEDING, A Parent's Guide* acknowledges those challenges and provides practical advice and workable solutions.

While many mothers and babies breastfeed without difficulty, others require assistance, especially in the early weeks. Fortunately, the breastfeeding problems featured in the media are rare, but serve to remind parents and professionals that breastfeeding is a learned skill that requires knowledge and support. While *Breastfeeding, A Parent's Guide* provides the knowledge base, parents must look to their health care providers for support. So keep this book handy and don't hesitate to ask your doctor, midwife, lactation consultant, or nurse for help.

I am grateful to the many parents who have shared with me one of the most intimate experiences of their lives, breastfeeding their baby. I hope that they have learned as much from me as I have learned from them.

Amy Spangler

Introduction

One of the most important choices you will need to make as new parents is whether to breastfeed or bottle-feed your baby. While the benefits of breastfeeding for both mother and baby are quite clear, the choice to breastfeed, as well as breastfeeding success, requires knowledge and support. A clear understanding of how the process works, and knowledge of how to manage problems that can occur are helpful. However, encouragement and support seem to be the keys to success.

Most physicians and parents agree that breastfeeding is the best method of infant feeding, yet many parents choose to bottle-feed their babies or stop breastfeeding after a brief period of time. Frequently their choice is based upon too little information, incorrect information, or too little support. *Amy Spangler's BREASTFEEDING, A Parent's Guide* is a wonderful resource for breastfeeding parents. It is a practical step-by-step guide to breastfeeding. It deals honestly and directly with the advantages as well as the concerns. The review of milk production is simple, yet complete and gives the reader a clear understanding of this natural process. The suggestions for beginning to breastfeed provide recommendations that can be changed to meet the needs of each mother and baby. The discussions of possible problems, special situations, and common questions answer nearly all of the concerns expressed by new parents.

The information found throughout this book, appropriate medical advice, and encouragement and support from someone they trust will help those parents who choose to breastfeed, breastfeed successfully and encourage those who are undecided to seriously consider breastfeeding.

Richard Bucciarelli, M.D.
Professor of Pediatrics
Associate Chairman, Department of Pediatrics
Chief of Division of Neonatology
University of Florida
Gainesville, Florida

What Does It Mean?

This book is intended for new and expectant parents, so there are very few medical terms used throughout the text. However, it is hard to talk about breastfeeding without using a few medical words. To increase your understanding as you read, you may find the following definitions helpful.

Afterbirth Pains: Afterbirth pains are uterine contractions that occur the first 3–5 days after birth while breastfeeding.

Alveoli: Alveoli are grape-like clusters of cells inside the breast that produce human milk.

Areola: The areola is the dark part of the breast around the nipple.

Colostrum: Colostrum is the first milk produced in the breasts. This thick, yellow fluid is produced during the last weeks of pregnancy and the first 3–5 days after birth.

Ducts: Ducts are small tubes that carry milk from the alveoli to the milk sinuses.

Mastitis: Mastitis is an infection in the breast. Signs of mastitis include flu-like symptoms, fever, pain, and redness.

Meconium: Meconium is a black, sticky material found in the lower bowel of newborns.

Milk Sinuses: Milk sinuses are small balloon-like sacs where newly produced milk is stored. Milk sinuses are located under the areola and drain to the outside of the breast through openings in the nipple.

Montgomery Glands: Montgomery glands are small pimple-like bumps in the areola, the dark part of the breast around the nipple. These small glands produce an oily material that helps to keep the nipples and the areolas clean and moist.

Oxytocin: Oxytocin is a hormone produced in the brain that causes the uterus and the small muscles around the milk-producing cells (alveoli) to contract.

Placenta: The placenta (afterbirth) is an organ inside the uterus that transfers nutrients from mother to baby during pregnancy.

Prolactin: Prolactin is a hormone produced in the brain that causes milk production.

Uterus: The uterus is a hollow, muscular organ where babies grow and develop during pregnancy.

Vagina: The vagina (birth canal) is the passageway that the baby goes through during birth.

Benefits of Breastfeeding

Whether you plan to breastfeed or are uncertain,
you need to know how breastfeeding
benefits your baby, your partner, and you.

Benefits to Mother

PHYSICAL

- Women who breastfeed have less vaginal bleeding and less risk of hemor-rhage (excessive bleeding) after birth. Breastfeeding (infant suckling) causes the release of oxytocin, a hormone produced in the brain that makes the uterus contract. Uterine contractions limit the flow of blood from the uterus.

- Uterine contractions, caused by the oxytocin, return the uterus to its non-pregnant size sooner.

- Milk production requires 500–1000 calories a day.[1] One-half of the calo-ries comes from body fat stored during pregnancy. The remaining calo-ries come from foods eaten each day. Women who breastfeed lose preg-nancy weight more easily than women who formula-feed.[2] However, high calorie foods with no nutritional value should be avoided.[3]

- Breastfeeding reduces the risk of breast cancer in young women.[4, 5] The longer you breastfeed, the lower your risk. Women who breastfeed 2 years or more have the most protection.

- Breastfeeding reduces the risk of uterine cancer.[6] The risk is lowest in women who have breastfed recently and for longer periods of time. There is less protection after 55 years of age.

❧ Women who breastfeed are less likely to develop ovarian cancer.[7]

❧ Breastfeeding improves bone density and reduces the risk of hip fractures in older women.[8]

❧ *Full* or *nearly full* breastfeeding can reduce fertility and aid child spacing.

- Babies are *fully breastfed* when no other liquids or solid foods are given.
- Babies are *nearly fully breastfed* when most feedings (more than 85%) are breastfeedings and non-breastmilk substitutes are given rarely.[9]

❧ Breastfeeding requires no mixing, no measuring, and no clean-up, making nighttime feedings quick and easy.

SOCIAL

❧ Human milk is always available. It requires no sterilization or refrigeration.

❧ Breasts and babies are portable. Disposable diapers are available. Travel can be simple. With a little practice, mothers can breastfeed discreetly anywhere. Mothers who are shy or easily embarrassed might want to choose a quiet place where they will not be disturbed.

EMOTIONAL

❧ Breastfeeding promotes a special relationship between a mother and baby, a closeness that comes with time and touch, a bond that lasts forever.

❧ Breastfeeding provides an opportunity for mothers to rest during the day, something every new mother needs.

❧ With one hand free, breastfeeding allows a mother to share her time and attention with other children or take care of personal needs.

ECONOMIC

- Parents who breastfeed save more than $1000 (US) in infant feeding costs during the first year alone.[10]

- Breastfed babies have fewer illnesses, fewer doctor visits, and fewer hospitalizations. As a result, parents who breastfeed have lower health care costs.[11, 12, 13]

- Breastfed babies are healthier, even those in day care. As a result, parents working outside the home miss fewer days of work and lose less income.[14]

Benefits to Baby

PHYSICAL

- Human milk is nutritionally perfect for human infants. Human milk changes to meet the needs of a growing baby, something formula cannot do.[15]

- Human milk is readily available and requires no preparation, sterilization, or refrigeration. This is very important for mothers and infants in developing countries or in emergency situations where food supplies are limited or can spoil easily.

- Human milk is easily digested, so breastfed babies have less gas, colic, and spitting up.[16]

- Human milk contains important nutrients as well as special protective factors. This is nature's way of safeguarding the immature newborn against infections.[17]

- Breastfeeding lowers the risk of asthma, colic, food allergy, and eczema in infants with a family history of allergic disease.[18, 19, 20]

❧ Breastfed babies have less diarrhea.[21]

❧ Breastfed babies have fewer urinary tract infections.[22]

❧ Breastfed babies have fewer respiratory infections.[23]

❧ Breastfed babies have fewer ear infections.[24]

❧ Breastfed babies are less likely to develop chronic bowel diseases including ulcerative colitis, Crohn's disease, and celiac disease.[25, 26, 27]

❧ Breastfed babies are less likely to develop insulin dependent diabetes mellitus (IDDM).[28, 29]

❧ Breastfed babies are less likely to develop some childhood cancers, including leukemia and lymphoma.[30]

❧ Breastfeeding promotes nervous system development and increases intelligence quotient (IQ).[31, 32]

❧ Breastfeeding may reduce the risk of Sudden Infant Death Syndrome (SIDS), the leading cause of death in babies after one month of age.[33, 34, 35] To further reduce the risk of SIDS:

- Sleep your baby on his back; do not sleep your baby on his tummy or his side.

- Place your baby at the bottom or foot of the crib or cot; do not place your baby in the center or at the top or head of the bed.

- Use a lightweight cover or blanket; do not use a pillow, comforter, quilt, or duvet.

- Keep your baby comfortable; do not let your baby get too hot or too cold.

- Keep your baby in a smoke-free environment during pregnancy and at least during the first year of life.

When mothers and babies share the same bed, babies breastfeed more often and have fewer periods of deep sleep, which may decrease the risk of SIDS.[36, 37] If you sleep with your baby, do not use a pillow, comforter, quilt, or duvet. Mothers who smoke or drink more than one serving of alcohol (beer, wine, liquor) a day should not sleep with their babies.

EMOTIONAL

❧ Breastfeeding gives babies a chance to touch, to smell, to hear, to see, to taste, to know their mothers from the first moment of birth.

COMMON CONCERNS

There are no disadvantages to breastfeeding. However, there are certain factors that some women find bothersome. As a result, some mothers choose to formula-feed or stop breastfeeding after a short period of time.

❧ Frequent breastfeedings may limit your freedom for the first 4–6 weeks while you are increasing your milk supply and learning to breastfeed. However, this gives you a chance to rest and to get to know your baby.

❧ Leaking can be annoying in the early weeks when babies are feeding at irregular times. However, leaking can be managed and is a good sign of milk production and milk release (see "Leaking," p. 80).

❧ Breastfeeding can be painful at the beginning of a feeding when the baby first latches on to the breast.[38] This is common. However, pain that lasts more than a minute or continues during the feeding or between feedings may be a sign of poor positioning or a breast infection. Breastfeeding should not be painful if the baby is positioned correctly on the breast (see "Milk Transfer," p. 30).

❧ The amount of milk taken at each feeding cannot be measured. However, frequent, watery stools (bowel movements) will let you know that your baby is getting enough to eat.

- Expect at least 3 stools a day for the first 3 days and at least 4 stools a day for the next 4 weeks.[39, 40]

- Your baby's stools will be sticky and black (meconium) for the first 1–2 days, soft and brown by day 3, and watery and yellow by day 4.

- Breastfed babies' stools look like a mixture of water, yellow mustard, cottage cheese, and sesame seeds!

- Expect small, frequent, watery stools with very little solid material. Sometimes, all you see is a yellow stain the size of your baby's fist.

- After the first 4–6 weeks, expect larger, softer, formed stools every 1–5 days.

🦋 Human milk is easily digested, causing loose, frequent, watery stools. However, there is little or no odor, which makes diapering more pleasant. This is important for dads who often have diaper duty!

🦋 Because human milk is easily digested, breastfed babies may feed more often and may not sleep through the night for several weeks or months. However, the same is true of many formula-fed babies. When your baby is 6–12 weeks old, you can begin to lengthen the nighttime sleep period if necessary. You can delay nighttime feedings by diapering, walking, and rocking.[41]

🦋 You do not need to follow a special diet while breastfeeding unless you have a family history of allergic disease or find that certain foods make your baby fussy (see "Breastfeeding the Baby with a Family History of Allergic Disease," p. 106). As long as you eat a variety of foods and drink to satisfy your thirst, both you and your baby will be fine. You will need to limit your intake of nicotine, alcohol, and caffeine.

🦋 Breastfeeding limits your choice of birth control. However, natural child spacing can be achieved with *full* or *nearly full* breastfeeding. This is called the Lactational Amenorrhea Method (LAM) of birth control.[42] For LAM to be effective, the following conditions must apply:

- You have had no menstrual period (monthly bleeding) since the birth of your baby.
- You breastfeed *fully* or *nearly fully*, giving juice, formula, or water rarely.
- Your baby breastfeeds at least every 4–6 hours day and night.
- Your baby is less than 6 months old.

When schedules or routines limit the frequency or length of breastfeedings or include frequent use of breastmilk substitutes, pregnancy is more likely. If pregnancy is not desired, another method of birth control is suggested. Choices include:

- natural family planning (sympto-thermal method)
- cervical cap
- female condom
- diaphragm
- intrauterine device (IUD)

- male condom
- spermicidal cream, foam, or jelly
- progestin implants (Norplant)
- progestin injections (Depo-Provera)
- progestin-only birth control pills

Combination birth control pills that contain estrogen and progestin are not recommended while breastfeeding.[43] Estrogen decreases milk production and can affect growth and development of babies. Birth control methods that contain only progestin are safe (Illustration 1).[44]

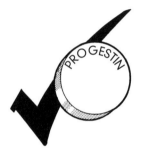 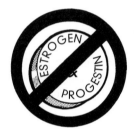

Illustration 1
Mothers who breastfeed should not take birth control pills that contain *estrogen.* However, birth control pills that contain *only progestin* are safe.

Some breastfeeding women have reported a decrease in milk supply when using progestin-only birth control methods. To limit this risk, delay the use of progestin-only methods until the baby is 6–12 weeks of age; then use progestin-only pills, which can be easily stopped if your milk supply decreases, rather than injections or implants.

Understanding Milk Production

The Structure and Function of the Human Breast

You may find breastfeeding easier and more effective if you know the different parts of the breast and understand how each part functions during lactation (milk production).

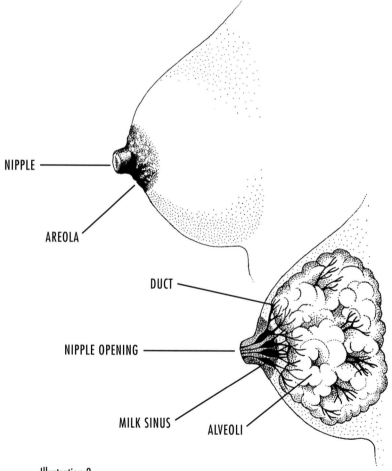

NIPPLE

AREOLA

DUCT

NIPPLE OPENING

MILK SINUS

ALVEOLI

Illustration 2
The human breast has many parts, each with a special function.

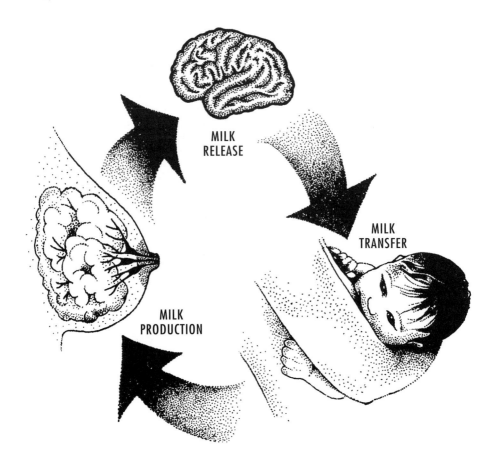

MILK RELEASE

MILK TRANSFER

MILK PRODUCTION

Illustration 3
To nourish a baby at the breast three things must happen: milk production, milk release, and milk transfer.

To nourish a baby at the breast three things must happen: milk production, milk release, and milk transfer. To accomplish these three things, you need a breast, a brain, and a baby (Illustration 3).

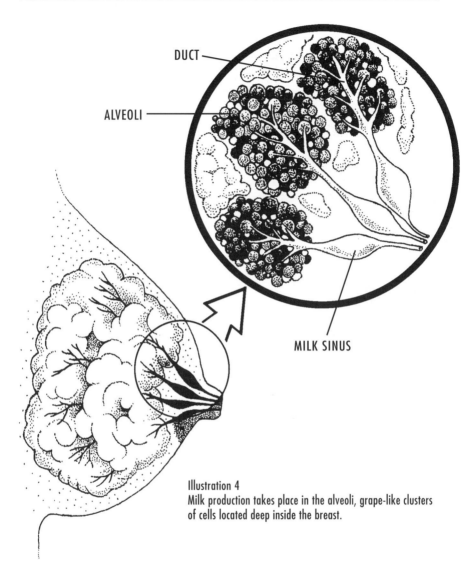

DUCT

ALVEOLI

MILK SINUS

Illustration 4
Milk production takes place in the alveoli, grape-like clusters
of cells located deep inside the breast.

Milk Production: Milk production takes place in the alveoli, grape-like
clusters of cells located deep inside the breast. The delivery of the
placenta (afterbirth) is the first stimulus for milk production, followed
by infant suckling or breastfeeding. Breastfeeding should begin as soon
as possible after birth, ideally within the first hour.[45, 46] The amount of
milk produced is determined by the amount of milk removed from the
breasts. Early, frequent breastfeedings, 8–12 feedings in a 24-hour
period, will usually produce a good supply of milk.[47, 48]

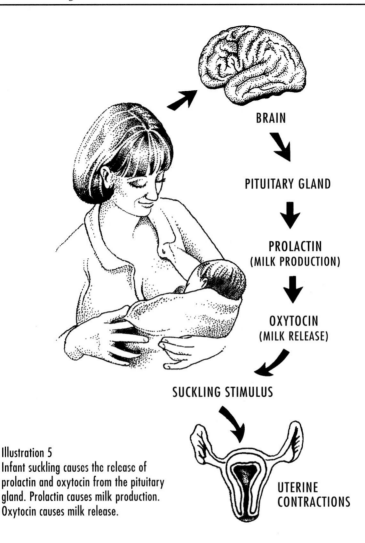

BRAIN

PITUITARY GLAND

PROLACTIN
(MILK PRODUCTION)

OXYTOCIN
(MILK RELEASE)

SUCKLING STIMULUS

UTERINE
CONTRACTIONS

Illustration 5
Infant suckling causes the release of
prolactin and oxytocin from the pituitary
gland. Prolactin causes milk production.
Oxytocin causes milk release.

Milk Release: When the infant begins to breastfeed, the following occur
(Illustration 5):

🐾 Suckling stimulates the nerves inside the nipple to send a message to
the brain.

🐾 The brain receives the message and signals the pituitary gland to
release two hormones, prolactin and oxytocin.

🌺 Prolactin causes the milk-producing cells (alveoli) in the breast to make milk.

🌺 Oxytocin causes the small muscles around each milk-producing cell to contract. Muscle contractions move the milk from the alveoli through a series of small tubes (ducts) into the milk sinuses, the small, balloon-like sacs located under the areola of the breast. During milk release, milk flows out from the milk sinuses through openings in the nipple.

This sudden release of milk from the breast is called the let-down reflex or milk-ejection reflex. It may take several seconds or several minutes for this release of milk to occur. It may also take several days or weeks for this reflex to develop fully. Many mothers have more than one let-down during each feeding. You may feel a tingling or burning sensation in the breasts when the milk lets down, or you may see milk leaking from one breast while the baby is feeding from the opposite breast. Don't be concerned if you feel or see nothing; every mother is different. Simply watch your baby. Look and listen for signs of swallowing. When your milk lets down, your baby's sucking pattern will change from short, rapid bursts of sucking to a slower, rhythmic, suckle-swallow pattern. The suckle-swallow pattern causes movement in the upper jaw which makes the baby look like he is wiggling his ears.

Oxytocin also makes the uterus contract, causing afterbirth pains. Uterine contractions occur while breastfeeding during the first 3–5 days after birth. They limit the flow of blood from the uterus and return the uterus to its non-pregnant size sooner.

Factors that can affect milk release include:

🌺 embarrassment

🌺 lack of confidence

🌺 lack of encouragement and support

🌺 pain

🌺 stress

🌺 tiredness

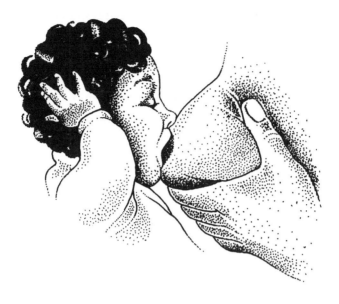

Illustration 6
To transfer (remove) milk from the breast, your baby must be positioned correctly.

If you are shy or easily embarrassed, choose a quiet place where you will not be disturbed. Nap when the baby naps, accept all offers of household help, and get encouragement and support from people you trust.

Milk Transfer (Removal): The more milk you remove from the breasts, through breastfeeding or milk expression, the more milk you will make. To remove milk from the breast, the baby must be positioned correctly on the breast and be able to coordinate suckling, swallowing, and breathing.

When positioned correctly, your baby's head and chest should be facing the breast. His mouth should be opened wide. His tongue should be over his lower gum, between his lower lip and the breast. His lips should turn out like a fish and lie flat against the breast. His nose and cheeks should gently touch the breast. His chin should press firmly into the breast (Illustration 6).[50] You may see little or none of the areola. However, this will depend on the size of your areola and the size of your baby's mouth. If part of the areola is seen, you will often see more on the top, above your baby's lip, and less on the bottom.[51]

- Breastfeed at least 8–12 times in 24 hours, but remember that every baby is different. Some babies will breastfeed every 2–3 hours, day and night, while others will cluster-feed, breastfeeding every hour for 3–5 feedings, and sleeping 3–4 hours between clusters. Some babies will breastfeed for 10–15 minutes on each breast, some will breastfeed for 30–45 minutes on each breast, and others will breastfeed for 15–30 minutes on one breast only.

- During the first 4 weeks, if your baby does not demand or ask to eat at least 8–12 times in 24 hours, you will need to watch for early signs of hunger or light sleep such as wiggling, finger-sucking, lip-smacking, coughing, or yawning and offer the breast at those times.

- Breastfeed as long as the baby wishes on the first breast before offering the second breast. This is called baby-led feeding. Watch your baby, not the clock. When the baby stops suckling and swallowing or falls asleep at the first breast, break the suction, burp him, wake him, and offer the second breast. If the baby breastfeeds poorly on the first breast, showing no sign of suckling and swallowing, offer the first breast again. Breastfeed well on one breast before you offer the second breast.[52, 53]

- Offer both breasts at every feeding, but do not be concerned if the baby seems satisfied with one breast. Each breast can provide a full meal. If necessary, hand express or pump the second breast to relieve fullness.

- Begin each feeding on the breast offered last.

Newly produced milk collects in the milk sinuses. When the baby is positioned correctly on the breast, the milk sinuses are drawn into the baby's mouth. With a wave-like movement of the baby's tongue, the milk sinuses are compressed between the roof of the mouth above and the tongue below. The action of the tongue, beginning at the tip, moves milk through the sinuses and out the openings in the nipple. When enough milk collects in the baby's mouth, a swallow occurs (Illustration 7).[49] Swallowing is one sign of milk transfer.

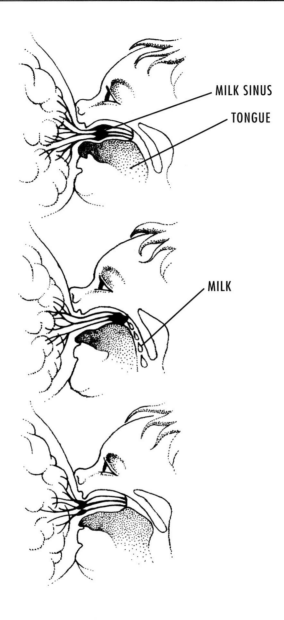

MILK SINUS

TONGUE

MILK

Illustration 7
When the baby is positioned correctly, the milk sinuses are compressed between the roof of the mouth above and the tongue below. A wave-like movement of the tongue moves milk through the sinuses and out the nipple openings.

Milk transfer is the key to effective breastfeeding. Some babies breastfeed often (8–12 times in 24 hours) but do not transfer (remove) milk from the breast. If you know the signs of milk transfer, you can be sure your baby is getting enough to eat:

- You hear or see your baby suckle and swallow while breastfeeding.

- Your baby has at least 3 stools and 3 wet diapers a day during the first 3 days and at least 4 stools and 6 wet diapers a day during the next 4 weeks.

- Your baby gains 4–8 ounces a week after the first or second week of life.

- Your baby loses less than 7% of his birth weight the first 5–7 days.

- Your baby is back to his birth weight by 14 days.

- Your breasts feel full and firm before you breastfeed and softer after you breastfeed.

- You see milk leaking from one breast while the baby breastfeeds from the opposite breast.

MILK COMPOSITION

There are three types of human milk: colostrum, transitional milk, and mature milk. Although each contains similar nutrients, they vary in content and volume. From 0–5 days after birth, colostrum is produced; from 5–15 days, transitional milk is produced; after 15 days, mature milk is produced. This change is gradual and may occur unnoticed. The rate of change may vary depending upon which pregnancy this is for the mother.[54]

Colostrum is a thick, yellow fluid. It is present during the last weeks of pregnancy and the first days after birth. Most mothers produce 1–3 ounces (30–100 ml) of colostrum a day. Small feedings of $1/4$–$1/2$ ounce (7–30 ml) during the first 2–3 days make it easier for your baby to adjust to life outside the uterus. Because these early feedings are small, some babies may seem hungry after breastfeeding and may *demand* or *ask* to breastfeed every hour. Supplements are seldom necessary unless the baby loses more than 7% of his birth weight. Colostrum is high in protein, low in fat, and rich in antibodies that protect babies from infection. Colostrum also causes bowel movements in the newborn, which help to remove meconium. Meconium is a thick, black, sticky substance that contains bilirubin. It is found in the lower bowel of newborns. When bilirubin levels increase, jaundice occurs. Early passage of meconium decreases bilirubin levels and limits jaundice in the newborn.

The content and volume of transitional milk changes gradually over a 10–15 day period. The rate of change is often slower in first time mothers. While sugar, fat, and calories in the milk increase, protein and antibodies decrease, until the levels of mature milk are reached.

Mature milk has two parts, hindmilk and foremilk. Foremilk or *first milk* collects in the milk sinuses. Foremilk is high in protein, low in fat, and low in calories, giving it a thin, watery appearance. Hindmilk or *behind milk* collects in the milk-producing cells or alveoli. Hindmilk is high in protein, high in fat, and high in calories, giving it a thick, creamy look. Foremilk is obtained at the beginning of a feeding, while hindmilk is obtained at the end of a feeding (Illustration 8). Hindmilk contains the fat and calories necessary for the rapid growth of newborns. When breastfeeding routines limit the length of feedings (mother-led feeding), babies do not get enough hindmilk or calories. To prevent this, breastfeed as long as the baby wishes on the first breast (baby-led feeding) before offering the second breast.[53] When the baby stops suckling or falls asleep at the first breast, break the suction, burp him, and offer the second breast. If he breastfeeds poorly on the first breast, showing no signs of suckling and swallowing, put him back on the first breast before offering the second breast.

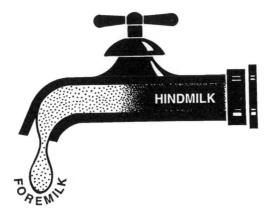

Illustration 8
Foremilk is obtained at the beginning of a feeding and hindmilk
is obtained at the end of a feeding. Hindmilk contains more of
the fat and calories babies need to grow. If you limit the length
of breastfeedings, babies get little or no hindmilk.

Prenatal Hand Expression

Colostrum collects in the breasts during the last weeks of pregnancy.
Removal of colostrum from the breasts during pregnancy is not recommended. Hand expression or any manner of pumping the breasts can
produce a breast infection or uterine contractions. Because uterine
contractions can cause premature labor, any possible benefit of prenatal
expression is outweighed by the likely risks.[55]

Preparing the Breasts for Breastfeeding

Frequently women worry that the size and shape of their breasts will affect their ability to produce milk. Fat deposits determine breast size and shape. While fat deposits protect the milk-producing cells in your breast, they do not affect your ability to produce milk. However, nipple size and shape can make breastfeeding easier or harder.

The Pinch Test (Illustration 9) will help you decide if your nipples are normal, flat, or inverted (Illustration 10). Do the Pinch Test on each nipple early in your pregnancy.

- Place your thumb and first finger at the base of the nipple near the edge of the areola.

- Press your thumb and finger together.

- A normal nipple will protrude or come out.

- A flat or inverted nipple will retract or sink in (truly inverted nipples are rare).

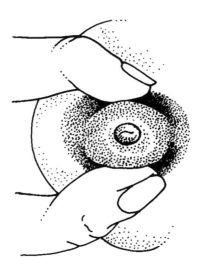

Illustration 9
The Pinch Test will help you see if your nipples are flat or inverted.

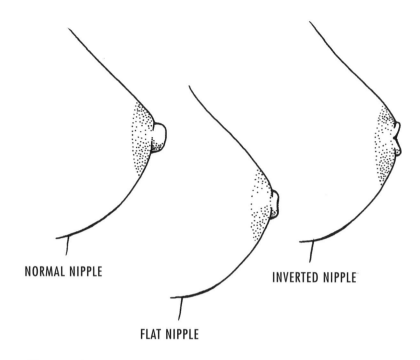

Illustration 10
Breast nipples come in all shapes and sizes and can make breastfeeding easier or harder.

If you see little or no movement of the nipple when you do the Pinch Test, put ice on the nipple for a few seconds. Remember, a flat nipple will show little or no movement; an inverted nipple will sink in, like a dimple; a normal nipple will poke out.

Flat or Inverted Nipple Treatment

Breasts come in all shapes and sizes, and most babies will learn to breastfeed on the breast at hand. Some women choose to wear breast shells during pregnancy to treat flat or inverted nipples, but research shows that breast shells are seldom helpful and may do more harm than good.[56] In addition, some women find the shells painful or embarrassing and prefer to wait until after the baby is born to see if he has difficulty with latch-on.

If you find that your baby is unable to grasp the breast and maintain a good latch, a breast pump can be used before each breastfeeding to gently pull the nipple out. Choose a hand pump, battery-operated pump, or electric pump, whichever is available. Adjust the suction control to the lowest setting, center your nipple in the opening (flange), and apply gentle suction for several seconds. If necessary, release the suction and repeat the action. As soon as the nipple comes out, remove the pump and quickly put the baby on the breast (see "Beginning to Breastfeed," p. 45).

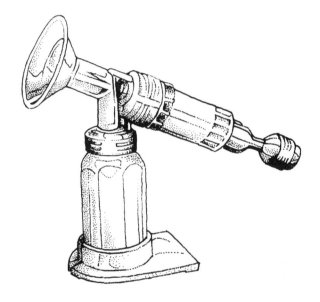

Illustration 11
A breast pump can be used before each breastfeeding to pull out flat or inverted nipples.
(Example shown is a manual pump by Medela®.)

BREAST SHELLS

A breast shell is a two-piece glass or plastic device that applies constant, even pressure to the areola, forcing the nipple through the center opening in the shell (Illustration 12). Do not confuse a breast shell with a rubber or silicone nipple shield (Illustration 13).

During the last weeks of your pregnancy, begin by wearing the shells for an hour or two each day. A snug bra will keep the shells in place. Slowly increase the time until the shells are worn 8–10 hours a day. To keep moisture from damaging your nipples, remove the shells every 2–3 hours and let your breasts air dry.

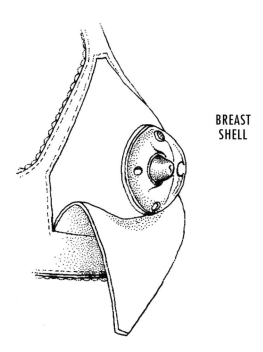

BREAST
SHELL

Illustration 12
Breast shells can be used during pregnancy to treat flat or inverted nipples.

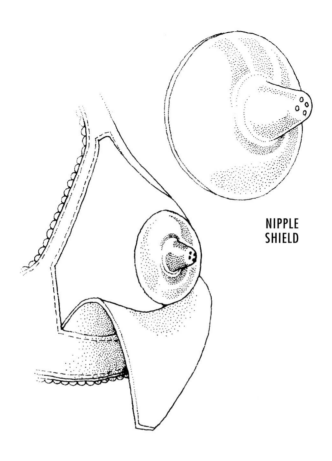

**NIPPLE
SHIELD**

Illustration 13
Rubber or silicone nipples shields are different from plastic breast shells. A nipple
shield can make latch-on easier when a mother has a flat or inverted nipple.
However, a nipple shield can limit milk production, milk release, and milk transfer.

NIPPLE SHIELDS

While the use of nipple shields may make latch-on easier, nipple shields can interfere with nipple stimulation, causing a decrease in milk production, milk release, and milk transfer (Illustration 13). Nipple shields should only be used with the guidance of a lactation consultant, doctor, or nurse, and only for short periods of time.[57] Some women use a nipple shield at the beginning of a feeding to aid latch-on and remove the shield when let-down occurs. If you are using a nipple shield, you need to check your baby's weight at least once a week.

NIPPLE EXERCISES

Many books recommend nipple exercises (nipple pulling and rolling) or other forms of nipple preparation (rubbing the nipples with a towel or washcloth) during pregnancy. However, nipple exercises or any form of nipple stimulation can cause uterine contractions and premature labor. Both the benefits and the risks must be carefully considered. Nipple exercises or other forms of nipple preparation do not prevent tender, painful nipples in the early weeks of breastfeeding.[58, 59] Correct positioning of the baby on the breast seems to be the important factor affecting nipple pain.[60]

Women who plan to breastfeed but who are uncomfortable touching their breasts might want to follow the simple suggestions for "Prenatal Breast and Nipple Care," p. 43.

Prenatal and Postpartum Breast and Nipple Care

Prenatal Breast and Nipple Care

❧ To prevent unnecessary drying, wash your breasts once a day using only clear water. The Montgomery glands, small pimple-like bumps in the areola (the dark part of the breast around the nipple) produce an oily material that keeps the nipples and areolas clean and moist (Illustration 2).

❧ If your nipple(s) are very dry, an unscented cream or lotion can be used. Use only a small amount. A little bit goes a long way.

❧ Expose your breasts to air and sunlight each day, if possible. Be careful to avoid sunburn.

❧ Remove your bra for a period of time each day and allow your clothing to gently rub against your nipples. If you prefer, wear a nursing bra and release the flaps, or cut a small hole in the center of a regular bra.*

*You do not need to wear a bra while you are pregnant or breastfeeding. However, if you prefer to wear a bra, you may find a nursing bra handy. For a proper fit, wait until the last weeks of your pregnancy. Choose a comfortable bra with cotton cups, adjustable straps, and simple flap fasteners. Avoid bras with underwires or bras that are too tight or bind, making it difficult to remove milk from all parts of the breast. If you prefer a bra with underwires, remove the bra for 1 or 2 feedings during the day and at night. Remove your bra at bedtime, unless you are leaking and need to wear breast pads.

Postpartum Breast and Nipple Care

❧ Use only clear water when you wash your breasts. Wash infrequently to avoid unnecessary drying.

❧ Limit the use of soaps, creams, lotions, and oils (Illustration 14).

❧ Whenever possible, air dry your nipples after each breastfeeding. Do not use hair dryers; quick drying, even with cool air, can damage your skin.

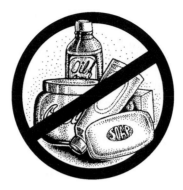

Illustration 14
Limit the use of soaps, creams, lotions, and oils on the breast while breastfeeding.

❧ Change breast pads frequently. Do not use pads with plastic liners.

❧ If your nipples are sore, put a few drops of colostrum or breastmilk on the areola and nipple after each breastfeeding until the soreness improves (Illustration 15).

❧ If your nipples become cracked or bleed, put a small amount of modified lanolin* on the damaged area after each breastfeeding to aid healing.[61]

*Modified lanolin, Lansinoh®, is a purified form of lanolin. It contains less pesticide residue and free lanolin alcohol than other lanolin products, making it safe for mothers and babies.

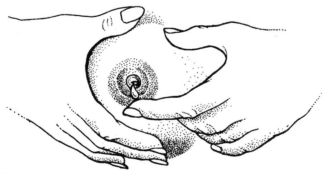

Illustration 15
Put a small amount of colostrum or breastmilk on the nipple and areola after each breastfeeding to ease soreness.

Beginning to Breastfeed

Your Baby's First Breastfeeding

- **Breastfeed as soon as possible after birth.** If the condition of mother and baby permits, breastfeeding should begin within the first hour, when babies are quiet and alert.[45] This first breastfeeding is a learning experience for you and your baby, so relax and enjoy this time together. Many babies are content to lick, nuzzle, and cuddle, safe and secure against their mothers' breast. Others will latch on and actively suckle if given the chance. Every baby is different.

- **Keep your baby with you day and night.** Mothers and babies should stay together (rooming-in 24 hours a day) whenever possible.[62] Rooming-in gives you and your baby a chance to get to know one another and gives you the opportunity to practice important parenting skills.

- **Delay unnecessary tasks.** When your baby's first breastfeeding is delayed, breastfeeding may be more difficult.[45] If possible, avoid all unnecessary tasks such as diapering, bathing, weighing, and measuring for at least 1–2 hours after birth.

- **Choose a comfortable position.** Choose a breastfeeding position that is comfortable for you and your baby (Illustration 16). Turn your baby on his side or tuck him under your arm so that his head and chest are facing your breast. Using pillows for comfort and support, place your baby at the level of your breast.

- **Support your breast.** If necessary, support your breast with your hand (Illustration 17). Place your thumb and fingers opposite one another on the breast, so that you can gently compress or shape the breast, making latch-on easier. Women with large hands and small breasts may prefer the *V-hold* or *scissors hold*. If you choose the *V-hold*, make sure you place your fingers outside the areola. Adjust the position of your thumb and fingers on the breast so that the shaped breast lines up with the widest part of the baby's mouth. For example, a mother using the *cradle position* (baby lying on his side and facing the breast) would shape the breast using a *C-hold*; while a mother using the *football position* (baby sitting up and facing the breast) would shape the breast using a *U-hold* (Illustration 17).

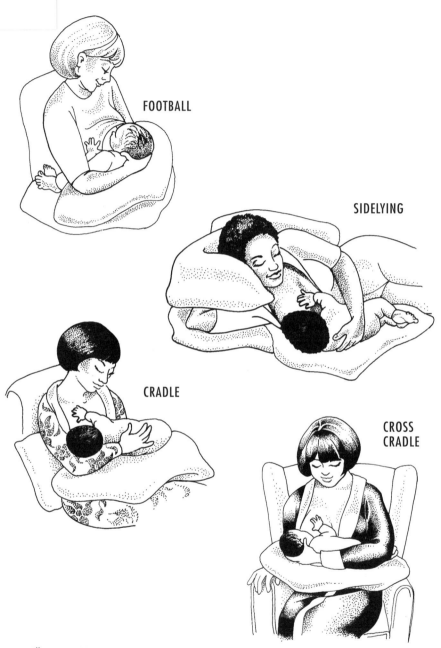

FOOTBALL

SIDELYING

CRADLE

CROSS CRADLE

Illustration 16
Choose a breastfeeding position that is comfortable for you and your baby. Use several different breastfeeding positions each day.

❧ **Express a few drops of colostrum.** Express a few drops of colostrum before you offer the breast. This will encourage the baby to latch on if colostrum is readily available.

❧ **Tickle your baby's upper and lower lips with your nipple.** Using the baby's rooting reflex, gently rub the baby's cheek closest to your breast with your finger or nipple. As he turns toward the breast, tickle his upper and lower lips with your nipple until his mouth opens wide.

❧ **Place your baby on the breast quickly but gently.** Keeping the baby's head and shoulders in a straight line, position the baby's lower lip against your breast and quickly but gently bring the baby forward and onto the breast.[51] Your nipple will point slightly toward the roof of the baby's mouth. Do not lean forward. Bring the baby to you. When positioned correctly, your baby's tongue should

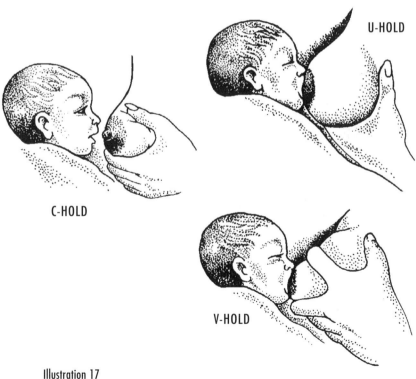

U-HOLD

C-HOLD

V-HOLD

Illustration 17
Place your thumb and fingers outside the areola to support and shape your breast.

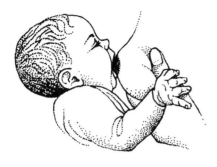
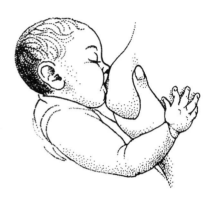

Illustration 18
Position your baby correctly on the breast.

be over his lower gum between his lower lip and the breast. His lips should turn out, like a fish, and lie flat against the breast. His nose and cheeks should gently touch the breast. His chin should press firmly into the breast (Illustration 18). Hold the baby close. This will prevent unnecessary pulling on the breast and keep the baby positioned correctly.

❧ **Check your areola.** When your baby is positioned correctly on the breast, you may see little or none of the areola. This will depend on the size of your areola and the size of your baby's mouth. You may notice that he is slightly off-center on the breast. As a result, you may see more areola on the top, above the lip, and less areola on the bottom.[51]

❧ **Check your baby's nose, cheeks, and chin.** Your baby's nose and cheeks should gently touch the breast. His chin should press firmly into the breast (Illustration 18). Support his shoulders and back with your hand; place your thumb and fingers below his ears and around his neck. Babies breathe through their noses. If you place your hand on the back of his head, you may press his nose into the breast and make breathing difficult. Women with large breasts can lift up gently on the breast with their fingers below or place a rolled washcloth under the breast to let air enter the nose. Do not press down on the breast with your thumb above or your nipple may slip out of the baby's mouth.

☞ **Watch your baby, not the clock.** When your baby stops suckling and swallowing or falls asleep at the first breast, break the suction, burp him, wake him, and offer the second breast.

☞ **Break the suction.** If your baby falls asleep at the breast and does not let go, you can break the suction by gently sliding your finger between his gums and into his mouth. Protect your nipple with your finger as you take the baby off the breast (Illustration 19). You may prefer to break the suction by pressing on the breast near your baby's mouth, making a small dimple with your finger (Illustration 19).

☞ **Breastfeeding should not be painful.** Breastfeeding should not be painful if the baby is positioned correctly on the breast. You might feel soreness when the baby first latches on. However, the soreness should stop as he draws the nipple and surrounding breast tissue into his mouth. If the soreness continues, remove the baby from the breast and try again.

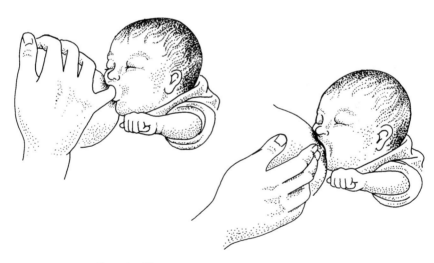

Illustration 19
Break the suction before removing your baby from the breast.

Your Baby's Next Breastfeedings

Keep your baby with you day and night. It may be several hours before your baby wakes to breastfeed again. While many babies breastfeed soon and often, others show little interest at first. Keep your baby with you day and night while you are in the hospital and during the first 2–4 weeks at home. Watch for early signs of hunger or light sleep such as wiggling, lip-smacking, finger-sucking, coughing, or yawning, and offer the breast at those times.

Breastfeed at least 8–12 times in 24 hours. The amount of colostrum taken during these early feedings is small (2–6 teaspoons), so your baby may seem hungry after feeding and may demand or ask to breastfeed every hour. Frequent breastfeedings give you and your baby a chance to practice this important skill while there is help available. Breastfeed at least 8–12 times in 24 hours. Expect to breastfeed every 1–3 hours during the day and every 2–3 hours at night, but remember that every baby is different. Some babies will breastfeed every 2–3 hours, day and night, while others will cluster-feed, breastfeeding every hour for 3–5 feedings and sleeping 3–4 hours between clusters.

Wake a sleepy baby. Sometimes a sleepy baby will not demand or ask to eat often enough. If you have a sleepy baby, keep him with you day and night. Watch for early signs of hunger or light sleep such as wiggling, lip-smacking, finger-sucking, coughing, or yawning, and offer the breast at those times. Additional suggestions for waking a sleepy baby include:

- dimming the lights
- removing his blankets or covers
- changing his diaper
- washing his bottom with a cool washcloth
- massaging his feet
- placing him in your lap in a sitting position, supporting his chin in one hand, massaging his back with the other hand

❧ **Relieve fullness and prevent engorgement.** Your milk supply will increase significantly 3–5 days after birth. Your breasts may feel firm and full. Frequent breastfeedings will relieve fullness and prevent engorgement. Breastfeed at least 8–12 times in 24 hours or every 1–3 hours. Offer both breasts at every feeding, but do not be concerned if your baby seems satisfied with one breast. If necessary, hand express or pump to soften the breasts and relieve fullness.

❧ **Position your baby correctly on the breast.** Breastfeeding should not be painful if your baby is positioned correctly on the breast. You might feel soreness when the baby first latches on. However, the soreness should stop as he draws the nipple and surrounding breast tissue into his mouth. If the soreness continues, remove the baby from the breast and try again. When your baby is positioned correctly, his head and chest should be facing the breast. His mouth should be opened wide. His tongue should be over his lower gum, between his lower lip and the breast. His lips should turn out, like a fish, and lie flat against the breast. His nose and cheeks should gently touch the breast. His chin should press firmly into the breast (Illustration 18). You may see little or none of the areola. However, this will depend on the size of your areola and the size of your baby's mouth.

❧ **Know the signs of poor latch-on.** To transfer milk, your baby must latch on the breast correctly. When positioned correctly, the nipple and the surrounding breast tissue should fill the baby's mouth. The nipple should be at the back of the baby's mouth, with little or no pressure on the nipple itself (Illustration 7). The nipple should look the same (smooth and round), before and after you breastfeed. When a baby is positioned incorrectly on the breast, nipple damage can occur. Signs of poor latch-on include:

- nipples that are flattened or creased after breastfeeding
- clicking sounds by the baby while breastfeeding
- dimpling of the baby's cheeks while breastfeeding
- pain while breastfeeding

❧ **Know the signs of milk transfer.** When positioned correctly, the milk sinuses, located beneath the areola, are drawn into the baby's mouth and compressed between the roof of the mouth above and the tongue below, forming a sandwich. A wave-like movement of the baby's tongue puts pressure on the milk sinuses, causing milk to flow out through the openings in the nipple (Illustration 7). A sudden release of milk from the breast is called the let-down reflex or milk-ejection reflex. You may feel a tingling or burning sensation in the breasts when the milk lets down or you may see milk leaking from one breast while the baby breastfeeds on the opposite breast. Don't be concerned if you see or feel nothing; every mother is different. Simply watch your baby. Look and listen for signs of swallowing. When your baby transfers milk, his sucking pattern will change from short, rapid sucks to a slower, rhythmic, suckle-swallow pattern. The suckle-swallow pattern causes movement in the upper jaw that makes the baby look like he is wiggling his ears.

❧ **Watch your baby, not the clock.** Breastfeed as long as your baby wishes on the first breast (baby-led feeding) before offering the second breast. When he stops suckling and swallowing or falls asleep at the first breast, break the suction, burp him, wake him, and offer the second breast. This will help to build a good milk supply and prevent breast fullness. Do not be concerned if your baby seems satisfied with one breast. Each breast can provide a full meal. If necessary, hand express or pump to relieve fullness in the second breast.

❧ **Break the suction.** Break the suction by gently sliding your finger between the baby's gums to the tip of your nipple (Illustration 19). Protect your nipple with your finger as you take the baby off the breast. You may prefer to break the suction by pressing on the breast near the baby's mouth, making a small dimple with your finger (Illustration 19).

❧ **Offer both breasts at each feeding.** Offer both breasts at each feeding, but do not be concerned if your baby seems satisfied with one breast. Begin each feeding on the breast offered last.

🐦 **Use more than one breastfeeding position each day.** Use moi⸳ ⸳⸳⸳⸳ one breastfeeding position each day (Illustration 16). Support your baby well in whatever positions you choose. This will prevent unnecessary pulling on the breast, keep the baby positioned correctly, and prevent nipple soreness.

🐦 **Keep a daily log.** During the first 2 weeks, while you and your baby are learning to breastfeed, you may want to keep a daily log of breastfeedings, wet diapers, and bowel movements (poops). As long as your baby has at least 8–12 breastfeedings, 6 wet diapers, and 3 poops a day, your breastmilk is all that he needs (see "Daily Log," p. 53)!

DAILY LOG

Day	8-12 Breastfeedings	6 Wet Diapers	3 Poops
(Sample)	⊪⊪ ⊪⊪ II	⊪⊪ I	III
Mon			
Tues			
Wed			
Thurs			
Fri			
Sat			
Sun			

Continuing to Breastfeed

The early weeks are a learning experience for the whole family, so relax and enjoy this time together. While a new mother can take care of herself and her baby, she should leave the household chores to others. Cobwebs can wait! Nap at least once a day when the baby naps, and wear your pajamas or nightgown during the first week as a reminder to family and friends that you are still recovering from the pregnancy, labor, and birth. The frustrations of parenting seem greater when parents are worn out from too little sleep. If necessary, limit visits and visitors. Continue to eat a variety of foods and drink to satisfy your thirst. You can begin light exercise 2–4 weeks after birth. However, listen to what your body tells you. Many mothers, eager to resume their active lifestyles, do too much too soon and quickly regret it.

As soon as your baby is breastfeeding well and gaining weight (4–8 ounces a week), about 4 weeks after birth, you can begin to let him set his own feeding schedule. Remember, every baby is different. Some babies will continue to breastfeed every 2–3 hours, day and night, for many weeks. Other babies will breastfeed every 1–2 hours when awake and sleep for longer periods of time. If your baby sleeps for 6 hours or more, you may need to express a small amount of milk to relieve fullness. Express only enough milk to relieve fullness and prevent engorgement. Do not express so much milk that you tell the breasts to keep making the same amount. Within 24–48 hours, your breasts will respond to your baby's changing needs and make just the right amount of milk.

Breastmilk is the only food your baby needs for the first 6 months of life.[63] During the second half of the first year, breastmilk remains an important part of your baby's diet along with iron-enriched solid foods. If breastmilk is not provided throughout the first year, iron-fortified infant formula is recommended. Cow's milk is not recommended until your baby is at least 1 year old.[64]

Breastfeeding provides benefits beyond the first year and should continue as long as the mother, father, and baby desire. Breastfeeding beyond the first year is common in many parts of the world. However, in some countries, breasts are seen first as sexual objects, and mothers who breastfeed in public or beyond the first year sometimes get dirty looks or nasty comments. As more women choose to breastfeed, breastfeeding will once again become the cultural norm, and individual attitudes will change. In the meantime, if you are shy or easily embarrassed, you might want to choose a private place where you will not be disturbed or wear loose clothing that makes discreet breastfeeding easy. However, if you choose to breastfeed openly and assert your right to do so, you will help to make it easier for other mothers. In some countries, laws protect a mother's right to breastfeed in public. Hopefully the day will come when nearly all women will choose to breastfeed and laws to protect their right to breastfeed will not be necessary. In the meantime, be confident in knowing that you are giving your baby the very best—nutritionally, immunologically, and emotionally.

Eating for Two

There are many questions that mothers have concerning nutrition during breastfeeding. How many calories should I eat while breastfeeding? How can I lose the extra weight I gained during my pregnancy? Are vitamin and mineral supplements necessary?

While some health care providers recommend a strict diet when breastfeeding, others suggest that mothers eat whatever they want. The following questions and answers may help you decide which foods are best for you and your baby.

Do I need to eat more calories while I am breastfeeding?

Nutritional needs vary with how much milk is produced. For example, the woman who supplements her baby with formula, in addition to breastfeeding, does not need as many calories as the woman who breastfeeds twins. Many nutritionists recommend 500 additional calories each day while breastfeeding. However, each woman's individual needs must be considered. Most women can produce enough milk while eating about the same number of calories as they did before they were pregnant. This way, some of the calories needed to make the milk are taken from fat stored during pregnancy.

The best recommendation is to eat to meet your appetite in the first month and try not to lose weight until your milk supply is well-established, about 4–6 weeks after birth. It is important to remember that the more you breastfeed, the more calories your body uses. The best weight loss is achieved when you breastfeed fully or nearly fully for 6 months.

How can I lose the extra weight I gained during my pregnancy?

Most women find they lose excess weight gained during pregnancy over a 6 month period. Although this may seem a slow rate of weight loss, restricting calories to lose weight more quickly is not recommended, since it can interfere with milk production. Although it can be argued that even malnourished mothers produce high quality milk, it is often at the expense of their own health. For example, if the mother does not eat enough calcium, her bones will be used as a source of calcium for her breastmilk and will become weakened as a result. By eating enough calories, you can be certain that other nutrient needs are met as well, including those for protein, vitamins, and minerals.

If you were *overweight prior to your pregnancy*, breastfeeding can help you lose weight. Once your milk supply is stable, 1,800 calories a day will maintain your milk supply and allow you to lose weight. If you engage in aerobic exercise or are very tall, you may need 2,000–2,400 calories a day. The best guide to use is the rate of weight loss. Women who are very overweight should not lose more than 4–6 pounds a month. Women who need to lose 20–25 pounds or less should not lose more than 3–4 pounds a month.

If you were *the right weight for height prior to pregnancy*, you will find that eating to meet your appetite and breastfeeding fully for 4–6 months will result in a gradual return to your pre-pregnancy weight. You may find that you will need to add calories to your diet as your baby reaches 4–6 months of age to keep from losing too much weight. It is important to remember that the minimum number of calories recommended is 1,800 calories. Again, women who engage in vigorous physical activity or are very tall may need 2,000–2,400 calories.

If you were *underweight prior to pregnancy*, you may need to add calories above your usual intake in order to keep from losing weight below what is right for you. This is especially important as the infant ages, if you are fully breastfeeding. Weight loss that results in a weight below your pre-pregnancy weight should be avoided while you are breastfeeding.

Do I need to drink extra fluid while I am breastfeeding?

Fluid intake is best regulated by thirst. In fact, excess fluids can actually decrease milk production! Many studies have looked at fluid intake and milk output and have found that the mother's thirst is the best guide. So follow your own thirst (about 6–8 glasses a day) and drink healthy beverages such as lowfat or nonfat milk, 100% fruit or vegetable juices, or water. Limit calorie containing beverages with little nutritional value (sodas, punch, alcoholic drinks) and non-calorie containing beverages (artifically sweetened "fruit" drinks and sugar-free sodas).

Do I need to take vitamin and mineral supplements while I am breastfeeding?

As long as you eat a balanced diet that includes a variety of foods, you do not need to take vitamin and mineral supplements. One supplement you may need while breastfeeding is iron. Many women do not menstruate (bleed each month) while fully breastfeeding, so your needs for iron and folic acid are less. However, extra iron is helpful in replacing the iron stores lost during pregnancy.

If you have iron deficiency or iron deficiency anemia, your doctor will prescribe an iron supplement (60–120 mg a day). Remember iron supplements are best absorbed on an empty stomach and should not be taken at the same time you take other nutrient supplements.

If you do not eat dairy products (due to lactose intolerance, vegetarianism, milk protein allergy, or dislike) *or other high calcium foods each day*, you should take a calcium supplement (600 mg of elemental calcium a day). Different forms of calcium have differing amounts of elemental calcium. Check the label and ask your pharmacist how much elemental calcium an individual supplement contains if you are unsure.

Dairy products are a source of vitamin D. *If you avoid dairy products and get less than 30 minutes of sun exposure a week*, you should take a vitamin D supplement (5–10 µg or 200–400 IU). The ultraviolet rays of the sun (with some help from the liver and kidneys) change a substance in the skin into vitamin D. Sunscreen blocks ultraviolet rays, so if you are depending on the sun for your vitamin D, wait 30 minutes before you apply sunscreen. If you are in the sun often, you can wait less than 30 minutes. Women who follow a strict vegetarian diet that does not include animal protein (meat, fish, eggs, or milk products) must choose foods carefully to get enough calories, protein, and nutrients, especially vitamin B_{12}, iron, vitamin D, and zinc. Protein and nutrients can be obtained by using soy products and by eating a variety of seeds, nuts, grains, legumes, vegetables, and cereals.

Will reduced fat and nonfat foods harm my milk?
Reduced fat and nonfat foods such as mayonnaise, cream cheese, salad dressings, cheese, etc. are not harmful. Be sure, however, to get some fat in your diet. If you are eating the minimum number of calories (1,800), your diet should include 60 grams of fat. This may seem like a lot, but it is not. Every animal product you eat except nonfat dairy products has fat. Lean chicken provides 2–3 grams of fat per ounce of meat, so it is very easy to get over 30 grams of fat from two small servings of meat a day.

What you eat determines the types of fatty acids in your milk. You may want to limit the amount of saturated fat (the type in animal products) by keeping your protein servings small and use mono- and polyunsaturated fats instead. You can easily do this by using a variety of oils, including olive, canola, sesame, corn, soybean, safflower, and walnut. If your diet does not supply fatty acids, the body substitutes different forms of fatty acids in your milk, so it is not wise to try to limit the fat too much. Instead, keep the added fats to 1–2 servings a meal and limit your animal protein intake to 2 servings a day.

Can I eat or drink caffeine-containing foods?

Small amounts (2–3 servings a day) of caffeine-containing foods are safe for breastfeeding mothers and healthy, full term babies. However, large amounts (5 or more servings a day) of caffeine-containing foods can cause fussy, wakeful babies. If you have a fussy baby, you might want to avoid or limit caffeine-containing foods such as coffee, tea, chocolate, and carbonated beverages.

Can I drink alcohol while breastfeeding?

Small, infrequent amounts of alcohol (2 ½ ounces of alcohol, 8 ounces of wine, or 24 ounces of beer) are safe.[65] However, alcohol can change the flavor of your milk, shorten your breastfeeding sessions, decrease your milk supply, and limit your baby's weight gain. Daily use of alcohol, even in small amounts, can affect your baby's motor development.[65] While small amounts of alcohol (1–2 drinks a day) are thought to be safe, 1–2 drinks can affect a mother's ability to care for her baby. To limit the effects of alcohol on you and your baby, drink no more than 1–2 drinks a week, and try not to breastfeed for at least 2 hours after you drink.

Can I use artificial sweeteners while I am breastfeeding?

Small amounts of artificial sweeteners are thought to be safe. Saccharin is a weak cancer-causing substance. The safe level of daily intake is 500 mg for children and 1,000 mg for adults. A popular brand of artificial sweetener using saccharin has about 14–20 mg per packet.

Aspartame is a combination of amino acids. Amino acids are what proteins are made from. Aspartame is concentrated and sweet and cannot be used by individuals with phenylketonuria (PKU). There is no proof that aspartame harms breastfed babies. However, you might want to limit your use of artificial sweeteners to 2–4 servings a day while you are breastfeeding.

Can I smoke while I am breastfeeding?

Smoking affects the breastfeeding mother and baby in many ways.[66, 67] It lowers the nutritional status of the mother, decreases the metabolism of vitamin B_{12}, alters zinc balance in the body, and lowers the levels of vitamin C and folic acid. Smoking causes a decrease in prolactin and oxytocin and a decrease in milk production, which can cause early weaning. Because the benefits of breastfeeding outweigh the risks of smoking, mothers who smoke are still encouraged to breastfeed. However, to limit the effects of smoking on your baby, smoke no more than 10 cigarettes a day and do not smoke in the house, the car, or near your baby.

How can I improve my diet to produce the highest quality milk possible?

- Eat the number of servings recommended (see "Suggested Breastfeeding Diet," p. 62).

- Eat a fish meal (especially cold water fish like salmon, mackerel, or bluefin tuna) 2–3 times a week.

- Use nonfat milk products and a variety of oils.

- Eat a minimum of 1,800 calories a day.

- Select foods that provide important nutrients (see "Nutrient-Dense Foods," p. 63).

SUGGESTED BREASTFEEDING DIET

FOOD GROUPS	NUMBER OF SERVINGS	EXAMPLES OF ONE SERVING
MILK/MILK PRODUCTS	3–4*	1 cup milk 1 cup yogurt 1 ½ cups cottage cheese 1 ½ ounces cheese 1 ½ cups ice cream
MEAT/MEAT SUBSTITUTES	2–3	2 ounces lean meat, fish, poultry 1 egg ½ cup cooked beans 2 tablespoons peanut butter 1 ounce cheese ½ cup tuna ½ cup nuts or seeds
CEREAL, BREAD, PASTA, RICE, LEGUMES	6–12	1 slice bread ½ roll, muffin, biscuit 1 tortilla ½ cup hot cereal ¾ cup cold cereal ½ cup rice, noodles, pasta
FRUITS/VEGETABLES	5–7	
Vitamin C	1	½ cup juice 1 medium orange ½ grapefruit ¾ cup cooked broccoli, bell pepper, cabbage

Vitamin A	1	1 cup raw or ½ cup cooked spinach,
		    broccoli, brussel sprouts, greens,
		    romaine lettuce
		½ cup apricots
		1 cup berries or melon

Others	3–5	½ cup fruit juice ¼ cup dried fruit 1 fresh medium fruit ½ cup raw vegetables
FATS, OILS, SWEETS	Limited amounts	1 teaspoon butter, mayonnaise, oil 1 tablespoon salad dressing 1 tablespoon sour cream

*Occasionally, something in the mother's diet will make a baby fussy. Foods which frequently cause fussiness include milk products, eggs, and nuts. If you have a family history of allergic disease or a very fussy baby, you might want to limit these foods in your diet as well as caffeine-containing foods such as coffee, tea, chocolate, and many carbonated beverages.

NUTRIENT-DENSE FOODS

FOLIC ACID	CALCIUM	VITAMIN C
leafy vegetables green beans legumes fortified cereals fruit	milk yogurt cheese sardines/salmon with bones dark green leafy vegetables dried beans and peas fortified orange juice fortified tortillas fortified tofu	citrus fruits and juices fortified juices strawberries broccoli cabbage potatoes green peppers

ZINC	VITAMIN A	VITAMIN B
beef poultry seafood eggs pork fortified cereals yogurt legumes seeds	dark green leafy vegetables orange/yellow vegetables liver egg yolk cheese milk butter	banana watermelon meat potatoes sweet potatoes nuts/seeds fortified cereals

Especially for Fathers

As a new father you will experience many feelings and emotions. Adjusting to fatherhood takes time, so be patient. Try to relax and enjoy each moment because it doesn't get any easier than this.

Breastfeeding is the best choice for every baby, and fathers benefit too! Happy, healthy babies need fewer doctor visits and fewer hospitalizations, making parenting easier. A breastfed baby, snug and content against your chest, gives you confidence in your ability to care for your baby. Nighttime feedings are simple when there is no formula to mix, measure, or warm. In addition, breastfed babies are portable, good news for active parents!

Breastfeeding is the natural way to feed your baby, but it does not always come naturally. Sometimes mother, father, and baby know just what to do, but more often they need to be taught. It will help to learn all that you can while you are pregnant. (Fathers are pregnant too!) This book will answer most of your questions, so be sure to read it carefully and keep it handy. Practice breastfeeding as often as you can while you are in the hospital. Keep your baby with you as much as possible and ask every question that comes to mind. Watch how the nurses help with breastfeeding and ask them to show you. Remember that mothers and babies need to breastfeed frequently and rest often. If necessary, limit the number of visitors and the length of visits. While some mothers are comfortable breastfeeding in front of family and friends (both male and female), many are not. It is important that a mother be relaxed. You know your partner best. So don't hesitate to speak up.

While it is nice to have help at home, family and friends can be a source of tension as well as a blessing if their knowledge of breastfeeding is limited. You may need to explain politely the benefits of breastfeeding, the importance of frequent feedings, feeding on demand, and nighttime feedings. Explain that it is better for mother and baby to nap during the day and breastfeed at night than for Grandma to bottle-feed the baby so mother can sleep through the night. Ask Grandma to take care of the home while your partner takes care of herself and the baby, but remember to tell Grandma how much you appreciate her help as you learn to be a father to her grandchild.

Breastfeeding is an important part of parenting, but equally important is the time you spend with your baby and the special moments you share. Find something that you enjoy doing with your baby and make it a routine. Taking walks, splashing in the tub, listening to music, playing games, or simply watching TV or reading the newspaper are ways for you and your baby to spend time together and to get to know one another.

Many parents ask, "When will things get back to normal?" The truth is, never! Your idea of "normal" will need to change. The two-seater sports car of your youth may no longer be practical, and minivans may look more appealing. You will need to adjust priorities and establish goals for a life that now includes another person. There may be little time at first for individual needs. However, as you learn to be a father to your baby, remember to be a friend and lover to your partner.

Despite all your efforts there will be times when things do not go well. Be prepared for the day when you arrive home from work to find your partner still in her nightgown. She and the baby are crying, the laundry needs to be done, and there is no dinner. Perhaps your day was just as bad! Instead of becoming angry, put a load of clothes in the washing machine, take the baby for a walk (it will relax all of you), order a pizza for dinner, and suggest that your partner make a cup of tea and take a warm bath. She will love you for understanding, and it will keep you both from saying things you might later regret.

Parenting is never easy, so relax and enjoy this time with your baby. Fathering a breastfed baby is a special joy, the benefits of which last a lifetime.

Managing Possible Problems

Breast Engorgement

SIGNS:

Breast engorgement often occurs 3–5 days after birth. The breasts are swollen, hard, and painful; the skin is red, shiny, and hot. Body temperature can increase slightly (to less than 100° F or 37.7° C).

CAUSE:

Breastmilk volume increases 3–5 days after birth, depending on which baby this is for the mother. The nutrients and fluid needed for milk production are carried to the breast through the blood and lymph system. When the fluid collects in the breast tissue, the breasts enlarge and swelling occurs. Early, frequent breastfeedings will relieve the swelling and soften the breasts. When feedings are infrequent, delayed, or missed, engorgement occurs.

RECOMMENDED TREATMENT:

- Put ice packs on your breasts between feedings. Bags of frozen peas wrapped in a wet washcloth work well. Some women use cold, raw cabbage leaves on the breasts after each feeding to relieve engorgement.*

  Why cabbage leaves relieve engorgement is unclear. There may be a substance in the leaves that decreases swelling or it may be the temperature of the leaves.68, 69 Rinse the leaves well in cold water before use. Place the leaves on the breasts with the nipples exposed until the leaves wilt. Apply fresh leaves only until the swelling decreases. Long-term use of cabbage leaves can reduce milk supply.

- Hand express or pump a small amount of milk or colostrum. This will soften the breasts and make it easier to position the baby correctly (see "Hand Expression," p. 122). If the breasts are leaking freely, a warm shower or tub bath or soaking the breasts in a pan of warm water may make milk expression easier. However, heat can increase swelling, so do not use warm water unless the breasts are leaking freely.

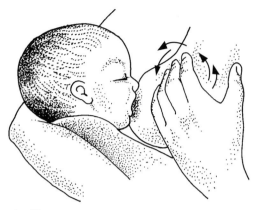

Illustration 20
Massage your breast to encourage the flow of milk and relieve fullness.

❧ Breastfeed every 1–3 hours during the day and every 2–3 hours at night. To increase the flow of milk, gently massage the breast in a circular pattern while the baby is breastfeeding, using the flat part of your hand (Illustration 20). If your breasts are still full and firm after feeding, hand express or pump to relieve fullness.

❧ Wear a bra for comfort and support. Avoid bras that are too tight or that bind, making it difficult to relieve fullness and soften the breasts. Avoid bras with underwires. If you prefer a bra with under-wires, remove the bra for 1–2 feedings during the day and at night.

A nipple shield may make latch-on easier. However, do not use a nipple shield without the guidance of a lactation consultant, doctor, or nurse. Nipple shields can decrease nipple stimulation, milk production, milk release, and milk transfer. If you use a nipple shield, check your baby's weight at least once a week.

TO PREVENT ENGORGEMENT:

❧ Breastfeed as soon as possible after birth.

❧ Breastfeed every 1–3 hours during the day and every 2–3 hours at night.

❧ Breastfeed as long as the baby wishes on the first breast before offering the second breast. If necessary, hand express or pump to relieve fullness in the second breast.

❧ Offer both breasts at every feeding.

❧ Begin each feeding on the breast offered last.

❧ If you delay or miss a feeding or the baby breastfeeds poorly, hand express or pump to relieve fullness.

Sore Nipples

SIGNS:

Breast or nipple soreness can occur during or between breastfeedings. Nipples are pink, red, or purple. Look for a break in the skin at the base of the nipple or on the top of the nipple. Thick, yellow material draining from the damaged area can be a sign of infection.

CAUSES:

Nipple soreness can occur during the first few days of breastfeeding. Soreness usually occurs at the beginning of a feeding when the baby latches on to the breast and draws the nipple and areola into his mouth. If the baby is positioned correctly on the breast, the soreness will only last a minute. If the baby is positioned incorrectly on the breast, the soreness will continue and nipple damage can occur. Other causes of nipple soreness include breast engorgement, breast infections, and the misuse of nipple shields, breast creams, or breast pumps.

RECOMMENDED TREATMENT:

❧ Position the baby correctly on the breast (Illustration 18). Turn your baby on his side or tuck him under your arm so that his head and chest are facing your breast. Use pillows to support the baby at the level of your breast. Tickle his upper and lower lips with your nipple until his mouth opens wide. Position the baby's lower lip against your breast and quickly but gently place the baby on the breast. Don't let him nibble his way on. Your nipple may point toward the roof of the baby's mouth. Do not lean forward. Bring the baby to you. His tongue should be over his lower gum, between his lower lip and the breast. His lips should turn out, like a fish, and lie flat against the breast. His chin should press firmly into the breast. His nose and cheeks should gently touch the breast.[51]

- If necessary, express a small amount of milk or colostrum to soften the breast before you allow the baby to latch on.

- Breastfeed on the least sore breast first. When a let-down reflex occurs and milk begins to flow, move the baby to the sore breast and breastfeed only long enough to relieve the fullness and soften the breast. If both breasts are sore, use a warm, wet washcloth and gentle massage to start the flow of milk before you put the baby on the breast.

- If necessary, limit the breastfeeding time on the sore breast and breastfeed more often, every 1–2 hours.

- Hold the baby close to prevent unnecessary pulling on the breast. Remember to break the suction before removing the baby from the breast.

- After each breastfeeding, put a small amount of colostrum or breast-milk on the areola and nipple of each breast (Illustration 15). Air dry nipples after each breastfeeding or dry gently with a soft cloth. Brisk rubbing with a towel or washcloth will increase soreness.

- Do not wash the nipples before each breastfeeding. Even water, used often, will dry the skin. Avoid soaps, creams, lotions, and oils (Illustration 14). If the nipples crack or bleed, put a small amount of modified lanolin on the damaged area after each breastfeeding to ease soreness and aid healing.

- If soreness, cracking, or bleeding continues, you can stop breast-feeding for 24 hours to let the nipple(s) heal. During this time you will need to hand express or pump to relieve fullness and feed your baby. If only one breast is sore, continue to breastfeed on the other breast.

✣ Thick, yellow material draining from the damaged area can be a sign of infection. You may need to rinse the area with a special solution and use an antibiotic cream or ointment. Call your doctor, lactation consultant, or nurse for help.

✣ A breast infection (mastitis) can occur when bacteria enter the breast through a break in the skin. Signs of infection include flu-like symptoms, pain, and fever. An antibiotic may be necessary. If signs of mastitis occur, call your doctor right away (see "Breast Infection (Mastitis)," p. 75).

✣ If necessary, take acetaminophen or ibuprofen for pain.

TO PREVENT SORE NIPPLES:

✣ Follow postpartum breast and nipple care suggestions, p. 43.

✣ Position the baby correctly on the breast. If necessary, hand express or pump to soften the breast and relieve fullness.

✣ Breastfeed as long as the baby wishes on the first breast before offering the second breast.

✣ Begin each feeding on the breast offered last.

✣ Breastfeed every 1–3 hours during the day and every 2–3 hours at night. If you delay or skip feedings, hand express or pump to relieve fullness.

✣ Use 2–3 different breastfeeding positions each day (Illustration 16).

✣ Break the suction before removing the baby from the breast (Illustration 19).

Blisters

SIGNS:

A collection of clear or bloody fluid underneath the skin.

CAUSE:

A blister can form on the nipple or areola of the breast. Blisters are caused by friction or pressure on the skin when the baby breastfeeds. Blisters are usually filled with clear fluid, but can be filled with blood. While the fluid can affect the taste of the milk, it will not hurt your baby. Because the fluid protects the new skin underneath, blisters should not be opened or drained. Leave them alone, and they will heal.

RECOMMENDED TREATMENT:

- To soften the blister and prevent cracking, put warm water on the blistered area before each breastfeeding, using a towel or washcloth.

- Position the baby correctly on the breast (Illustration 21).

- Avoid breastfeeding positions that put pressure on the blistered area.

- If necessary, begin each feeding on the breast without the blister. When a let-down reflex occurs and milk begins to drip, switch to the breast with the blister.

- If necessary, limit the feeding time on the breast with the blister and breastfeed more often, every 1–2 hours.

TO PREVENT BLISTERS:

- Position the baby correctly on the breast (Illustration 21). Tickle his upper and lower lips with your nipple until his mouth opens wide. Position the baby's lower lip against your breast and quickly but gently place the baby on the breast.

- Use 2–3 different breastfeeding positions each day (Illustration 16).

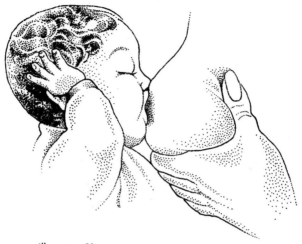

Illustration 21
When your baby is positioned correctly, his nose, cheeks,
and chin should touch the breast.

❧ Hold the baby close to prevent unnecessary pulling on the breast.

❧ Offer both breasts at every feeding. Do not be concerned if the baby seems satisfied with one breast. If necessary hand express or pump to relieve fullness in the second breast.

❧ Begin each feeding on the breast offered last.

Plugged Duct

SIGNS:

Signs of a plugged duct include a red, tender area or small lump in the breast. The area or lump may or may not be painful.

CAUSE:

Narrow tubes (ducts) carry milk from the alveoli to the milk sinuses. When feedings are delayed or missed, or when the baby breastfeeds poorly, milk can collect in the ducts and form a thick plug or small lump (Illustration 22).

RECOMMENDED TREATMENT:

- ❧ Put warm water on the plugged area before each breastfeeding.

- ❧ Breastfeed more often during the day.

- ❧ Begin each feeding on the breast with the plug.

- ❧ Adjust the position of the baby's mouth on the breast so that the baby's nose is pointing toward the plug.

- ❧ Gently massage the plugged area while the baby is feeding (Illustration 20).

- ❧ Hand express or pump after each breastfeeding to remove the plug and relieve fullness.

- ❧ Choose a breastfeeding position that best relieves fullness in the affected area.

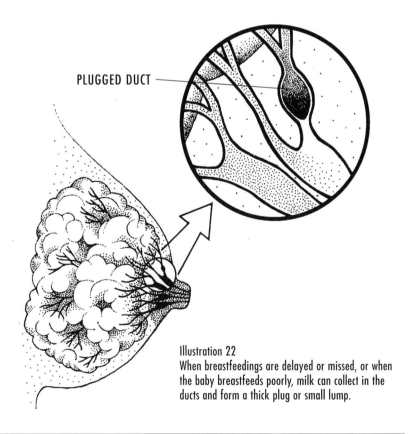

PLUGGED DUCT

Illustration 22
When breastfeedings are delayed or missed, or when the baby breastfeeds poorly, milk can collect in the ducts and form a thick plug or small lump.

TO PREVENT PLUGGED DUCTS:

❦ Position the baby correctly on the breast.

❦ Use 2–3 different breastfeeding positions each day.

❦ Do not delay or miss feedings.

❦ If necessary, pump or hand express to relieve fullness.

❦ Avoid bras that are too tight or that bind making it difficult to relieve fullness in all parts of the breast. Avoid bras with underwires. If you prefer a bra with underwires, remove the bra for 1–2 feedings during the day and at night.

Breast Infection (Mastitis)

SIGNS:

Women with a breast infection often describe flu-like symptoms, including weakness, headache, nausea, soreness, chills, and fever (greater than 101° F or 38.4° C). The breast can be red, hot, and painful.

CAUSE:

When breastfeedings are infrequent, delayed, or missed, or when babies are positioned incorrectly on the breast, milk collects in the breast and puts pressure on the surrounding tissue, causing engorgement. Engorgement damages the tissue and increases the risk of infection. When bacteria enter the breast through an opening in the nipple or a break in the skin, the damaged tissue becomes infected.

RECOMMENDED TREATMENT:

❦ Call your doctor. A prescription medicine (antibiotic) may be necessary. Although your symptoms may improve after 24–48 hours, take the medicine according to instructions until it is gone (usually 14 days).

✿ Put warm water on the infected area before each breastfeeding to aid let-down and relieve pain. Warm washcloths, a warm shower or tub bath, or soaking the breasts in a pan of warm water works well.

✿ Continue to breastfeed frequently on both breasts. The infection will not harm your baby. Breastfeed every 1–3 hours during the day and every 2–3 hours at night.

✿ Start each feeding on the uninfected breast until the let-down reflex occurs, then switch to the infected breast. Breastfeed only until the breast is soft. If necessary, hand express or pump to soften the breast and relieve fullness.

✿ You can apply cold packs after each breastfeeding to relieve pain and reduce swelling. Bags of frozen peas wrapped in a cold washcloth work well.

✿ Drink enough fluid to satisfy your thirst. Water and unsweetened fruit juices are best.

✿ Take acetaminophen or ibuprofen for pain.

✿ Get plenty of rest. To save time and energy, keep the baby close.

TO PREVENT A BREAST INFECTION:

✿ Position the baby correctly on the breast (Illustration 21).

✿ If you delay or miss a feeding or if the baby breastfeeds poorly, hand express or pump to soften the breasts and relieve fullness.

✿ Use 2–3 different breastfeeding positions each day (Illustration 16).

✿ Do not delay or miss feedings.

✿ Avoid bras that are too tight or that bind, making it difficult to relieve fullness in all parts of the breast. Avoid bras with underwires. If you prefer a bra with underwires, remove the bra for 1–2 feedings during the day and at night.

✿ Wean gradually. Pump or hand express to relieve fullness and soften the breasts.

Yeast-like Fungus Infections
(Thrush, Candidiasis, Moniliasis)

SIGNS:

Baby: The baby can become infected during vaginal birth or while breastfeeding. Signs of infection often appear 2–4 weeks after birth and include small white patches in the mouth (thrush) and a bright red rash in the diaper-area.

Mother: The mother can become infected while breastfeeding. Signs of infection include small red or white patches on the breast, red or purple nipples, and sharp, shooting pain in the breast. Frequently the breasts look normal and severe pain is the only symptom. Some women also have a thick, white vaginal discharge with redness, itching, and burning in the birth canal (vagina).

Father or sexual partner: Candida can spread easily from one family member to another through close contact. Your partner can become infected during sex. Signs of infection include a red rash on or around the penis and small white patches in the mouth.

CAUSE:

Candida is a yeast-like fungus that grows in dark, damp places. It can infect the birth canal, nipple, and breast of the mother as well as the mouth and diaper-area of the baby. Candida is found in the birth canal of most women; as a result, babies can become infected during vaginal birth. While the infection is not serious, it can be very painful. Sometimes a baby will refuse to breastfeed.

RECOMMENDED TREATMENT:

❧ Treat both mother and baby, even if only one has symptoms. This will prevent reinfection. You may need to call your doctor as well as your baby's doctor. Treat your sexual partner or any family member (siblings) with signs of infection.

Mother: Rinse the breasts with clear water after each breastfeeding. Your doctor will recommend one of the following medications:

Nystatin® (mycostatin), Monistat® (miconazole), or Lotrimin® (clotrima-zole). Put the ointment on the nipple and areola of both breasts after each breastfeeding for 14 days. If the pain is severe, use one of the above medications with cortisone (Mycolog®, Lotrisone®) for the first 1–3 days. Gently massage the medication into the nipples. It is not necessary to remove the ointment before breastfeeding.

Baby: Your baby's doctor will prescribe medication in liquid form, Nystatin® (mycostatin) for the baby's mouth, and in ointment form, Monistat® (miconazole) or Lotrimin® (clotrimazole), for the baby's diaper area. The ointment used on the mother's nipples also can be used on the baby's bottom. Paint the liquid on the inside of the baby's mouth (cheeks, gums, tongue, and roof) after each breastfeeding, using a clean cotton swab for each part of the mouth (Illustration 23). If you put a used cotton swab back into the medicine bottle, you can transfer the fungus from the baby's mouth to the bottle. Put the ointment on the red rash in the diaper area during each diaper change.

- Expose your breasts as well as the baby's bottom to air and sunlight. Be careful to avoid sunburn.

- Change breast pads and diapers frequently. Do not use pads with plastic liners.

- Boil all rubber nipples and pacifiers daily for 20 minutes. Replace with new ones after the first and second week of treatment.

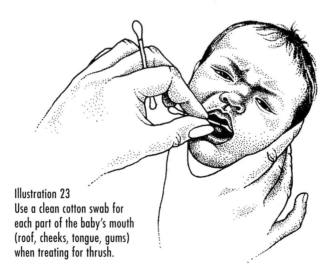

Illustration 23
Use a clean cotton swab for
each part of the baby's mouth
(roof, cheeks, tongue, gums)
when treating for thrush.

❧ Wash bras in hot, soapy water each day and rinse well. Boil all pump parts for 20 minutes each day.

❧ Wash your hands carefully before each breastfeeding and after each diaper change.

❧ Use condoms during sex. Do not let your partner's mouth come into contact with your breasts.

❧ If signs of infection remain after 14 days of treatment, the fungus may be resistant to the medicine in the ointment. You can choose a different ointment and treat for 4–6 weeks or apply a 1% solution of gentian violet once a day for 3 days. Using a cotton swab, paint the solution on the nipple and areola of both breasts and on the inside of the baby's mouth (cheeks, gums, tongue, and roof). The purple solution will stain the skin and clothing, so you might want to wear an old bra and tee-shirt.

❧ Resistant infections that do not respond to ointments or solutions can be treated with pills or tablets taken by mouth. Fluconazole is approved by the Food and Drug Administration (FDA) for use in adults and infants. However, fluconazole should only be used if topical treatments (ointments and solutions) fail to relieve symptoms. You will need to call your doctor for a prescription. In addition, you may want to avoid foods that support the growth of fungus, such as alcohol, sugar, dairy products, wheat, nuts, peanut butter, dried fruits, and fruit juices.

TO PREVENT YEAST-LIKE FUNGUS INFECTIONS:

❧ Wash your hands carefully before each breastfeeding and after each diaper change.

❧ Expose your breasts and your baby's bottom to air and sunlight whenever possible. Be careful to avoid sunburn.

❧ Change breast pads and diapers frequently. Do not use pads with plastic liners.

❧ Avoid the use of nipple creams and lotions, which may encourage the growth of yeast-like fungus or bacteria.

❧ Air dry nipples after each breastfeeding whenever possible.

Leaking

CAUSE:

Leaking often occurs during the early weeks when the baby is breast-feeding at irregular times. It may be 6–12 weeks before your baby has a regular feeding schedule. Until that time, your milk supply will continue to change. While leaking is normal, it does not occur in every mother. Leaking can occur when you think about your baby, when you hear your baby or another baby cry, when you delay or miss a feeding and your breasts overfill, or when you are making love and have an orgasm (sexual climax).

RECOMMENDED TREATMENT:

- To control leaking, press firmly against the nipple of each breast with the palm of your hand or your wrist or fold your arms tightly across your chest.

- Breast pads provide short-term protection and come in all shapes and sizes, disposable as well as reusable. You can even make your own pads using cloth diapers, cotton fabric, or men's handkerchiefs. Change pads frequently. Do not use pads with waterproof liners.

- Choose clothing with light colors and small prints that will cover up a multitude of mishaps.

- Breastfeed your baby before making love or going to bed. This will limit the amount of milk in the breasts and allow time for sex or sleep, whichever comes first!

Special Situations

Breastfeeding after Cesarean Birth

Cesarean birth is the surgical removal of the baby through an incision or opening made in the mother's abdomen. Nearly 20–30% of all births are cesarean births. Cesarean births are seldom planned; as a result, parents may experience many feelings including anger, relief, frustration, joy, and sadness. Discuss your feelings openly with your doctor, family, or friends. It may help to talk with other parents who have had an unplanned cesarean birth. While cesarean birth will not affect your ability to produce milk, pain and weakness may make it necessary for you to depend on others for help. If mother or baby need special care, the start of breastfeeding may be delayed.

IN THE HOSPITAL

Breastfeed as soon as possible after birth. If the start of breastfeeding is delayed for more than 24–48 hours, begin expressing your milk. Hand express or pump every 2–4 hours during the day and every 4–6 hours at night. An automatic, self-cycling electric breast pump with a double collection kit that lets you pump both breasts at the same time works best (Illustration 24). Set the suction control on the lowest setting and pump until the flow of milk or colostrum slows down (5–10 minutes), rest 3–5 minutes, and repeat once or twice. Pump each breast for a total of 15–20 minutes.

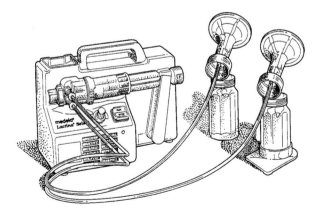

Illustration 24
An automatic self-cycling electric breast pump with a double collection kit lets you pump both breasts at the same time. (Example shown is a Lactina™ by Medela®.)

❧ Choose a comfortable position (Illustration 16) to breastfeed. Use extra pillows to protect the incision and provide support.

❧ Position the baby correctly on the breast (see "Beginning to Breastfeed," p. 45). You may need help with positioning, turning, and burping (babies born by cesarean birth often have more mucus).

❧ Breastfeed whenever the baby seems fussy or hungry or at least 8–12 times in 24 hours. Expect to breastfeed every 1–3 hours during the day and every 2–3 hours at night. Breastfeed as long as the baby wishes on the first breast before offering the second breast.

❧ Increase the amount of protein (meat, fish, milk, eggs, tofu) and fiber (whole grains, raw vegetables) in your diet.

❧ Drink to satisfy your thirst; warm liquids increase bowel and bladder activity.

❧ Take short, frequent walks; mild exercise increases bowel activity and helps mothers regain their strength.

❧ Get plenty of rest; limit phone calls and visitors.

❧ Pain medicine may be necessary for several days. Your doctor will order medicine that is safe for breastfeeding mothers and babies. To limit the effect of the medicine on the baby, take the medicine after you breastfeed.

AT HOME

❧ Breastfeed whenever the baby seems fussy or hungry or at least 8–12 times in 24 hours. Expect to breastfeed every 1–3 hours during the day and every 2–3 hours at night. Some babies will not ask or demand to eat often enough. Therefore, during the first 2–4 weeks, if your baby does not wake to feed, you may need to watch for early signs of hunger or light sleep, such as wiggling, finger sucking, lip smacking, coughing, or yawning and offer the breast at those times.

❧ Keep the baby in the room with you to save time and energy.

❧ Get plenty of rest. Nap when the baby naps.

❧ Limit your activity. Avoid heavy lifting, household chores, and brisk exercise for 4–6 weeks.

❧ To promote healing and speed recovery, continue:
  • high protein, high fiber diet
  • liquids to satisfy your thirst
  • mild to moderate exercise

Breastfeeding the Premature Baby

The birth of a tiny baby born weeks or months premature can be scary. Why did this happen? Was it something I did? Was it something I didn't do? Will he live? Will he be normal? How long will he be in the hospital? Can I hold him? How will he eat if he is too little to suck? Can I breastfeed?

Premature babies can be breastfed, even those needing special care. Breastfeeding gives parents a chance to share in the care of their baby, to do something that no one else can do, to parent in a very special way. If your baby is too small or too sick to breastfeed in the beginning, he can still be fed your breastmilk. When you give birth prematurely, your milk contains just the right amount of nutrients to meet your baby's needs. In addition, human milk contains special cells that protect babies against infections, which are common in premature babies.[70] Breastmilk is easy to digest, which is important for premature babies with immature digestive systems.[71] Also, research shows that premature babies who are fed human milk for at least the first month of life have a higher intelligence quotient (IQ) at age 7–8 years than babies fed infant formula.[72]

Let your baby's doctor and nurses know as soon as possible that you plan to breastfeed. The hospital staff can give you information on milk production as well as expression, collection, and storage of breastmilk. In addition, they can put you in touch with other parents who have breastfed premature babies. These parents, along with the medical team, can help you develop realistic goals and provide you with much needed encouragement and support.

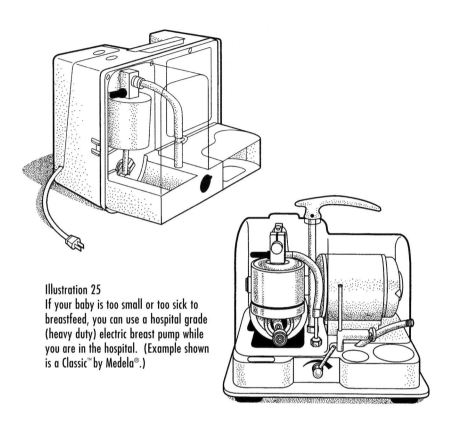

Illustration 25
If your baby is too small or too sick to breastfeed, you can use a hospital grade (heavy duty) electric breast pump while you are in the hospital. (Example shown is a Classic™ by Medela®.)

EARLY FEEDINGS

Your baby may be too small or too sick to breastfeed in the beginning and will need to be fed a special liquid through a small tube or needle that is placed in one of his veins (intravenous feeding). As his condition improves, he will be fed your breastmilk through a small tube that is passed through his nose into his stomach (gavage feeding).

PUMPING

- Begin pumping as soon as possible after birth. Unless you are very sick, it is important to start pumping within 24–48 hours. If your baby is too small or too sick to breastfeed, ask your nurse for a *hospital grade* electric breast pump to use while you are in the hospital (Illustration 25). Small electric, battery, or hand pumps are seldom adequate. When you go home, you can rent a *hospital grade* electric pump from the hospital, pump rental stations, drugstores, or a medical supply company. Check with your baby's doctor, lactation consultant, or nurse for the location nearest your home. Your expressed colostrum or breastmilk can be collected and fed to your baby or frozen and used later.

- Each time you pump and before you handle the pump parts, wash your hands with soap and water and rinse well.

- Put warm, wet washcloths on your breasts for 1–3 minutes.

- Gently massage your breasts using the flat part of your hand.

- Tickle your nipple with your finger. This will cause a let-down reflex and make milk expression easier.

- Relax and think about your baby. This will cause milk release and increase the amount of milk obtained.

- Moisten the pump horn (funnel) with water. Center your nipple in the opening.

- Set the suction control to the lowest setting and pump for 1–3 minutes. Slowly increase the pressure as long as you are comfortable.

- If you are pumping one breast at a time, pump for 5–10 minutes, switching to the opposite breast when the flow of colostrum or milk slows down. Pump each breast for a total of 15–20 minutes or until the breasts are soft and the flow of milk slows to a drip. The amount of milk you make will depend on the amount of milk you remove from the breasts. When the breasts stay full, your body will respond by making less milk (this is how mothers wean when their babies are older).

- Pump *at least* 5 times a day (for a total of 100 minutes). You will need to pump every 2–4 hours during the day and every 4--6 hours at night when awake. Once you learn to pump easily, you may want to double pump (pump both breasts at the same time). Pump for 5–10 minutes or until the flow of milk or colostrum slows down, rest for 3–5 minutes, then repeat once or twice. Double pumping increases prolactin levels, which increases milk production. In addition, double pumping saves time so you can spend more time with your baby. With double pumping, you may find that one breast softens before the other and that you still need to single pump and massage to relieve the fullness in the second breast. Many mothers pump every 3 hours during the day and sleep for 6 hours at night. Since pumps never get tired, hungry, or full, think of pumping as a special time to relax, think about your baby, and "feed" him. If you pump just before you go to bed, you will be able to sleep comfortably for a longer period of time. If you need to stop a pumping session before you are done, you can come back to it a short time later.

During the first week, as your breasts change from making colostrum to making mature milk, you may feel very full or engorged. You will need to pump more to relieve the fullness and stay comfortable. This will help you to build a good milk supply that can later adjust to your baby's needs as he grows. In the beginning, you may make more milk than your baby needs. However, if you do not relieve the fullness and soften your breasts, you may never have the full supply of milk that your baby will need later.

Your first attempts at pumping may only produce enough milk or colostrum to cover the bottom of the collection container. Don't get discouraged. It may take several days or weeks for you to see an increase in the amount of milk obtained. Like breastfeeding, pumping is a learned art. Many mothers get more milk with the first pumping session than with the next 3–4, and then the amount slowly increases for several days. If you are not getting at least 1 ounce per pumping session by the end of the first week, talk with the lactation consultant or your doctor about ways to increase your milk supply.

- ❧ Establish a routine — same time, same place. Choose a quiet, comfortable place where you will not be disturbed. If necessary, take the telephone off the hook and lock the door.

- ❧ Get organized and gather all of your supplies together. Include a healthy snack and drink for yourself.

⚘ Relax and think about your baby. Plan to do some relaxation exᵣᵣᵣᵢₛₑₛ at least once a day even if you cannot do them just before pumping.

⚘ Listen to a relaxation tape while pumping.[73]

⚘ Make a phone call to the nursery to check on your baby's condition.

⚘ Look at a picture of your baby or hold something he has worn.

⚘ If you are able to pump in the hospital, sit next to your baby's crib or isolette; hold his hand if possible.

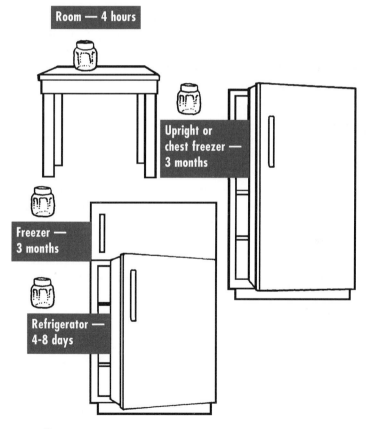

Illustration 26
Breastmilk storage recommendations for premature or sick babies.

❧ Put warm, wet washcloths on the breasts for 1–3 minutes before pumping, or plan to pump right after taking a bath or shower.

❧ Gently massage the breasts in a circular pattern using the flat part of your hand (Illustration 20).

❧ Roll your nipple between your finger and thumb to stimulate a let-down reflex.

❧ Do not use birth control pills that contain estrogen (Illustration 1). Delay the use of progestin-only birth control pills, injections, or implants for 6–12 weeks or until your milk supply is stable.

Put the expressed milk into sterile containers provided by the nursery. Glass or hard plastic containers with solid lids are recommended. Label each container with your baby's name, your name, the date, and the time. If you have taken any medicine within four hours of pumping, write the name of the medicine on the label. Ask your baby's nurse how much he is being fed every 24 hours and store your milk in 24 hour portions to prevent waste. It is best to provide fresh, unfrozen breastmilk each day if possible since freezing affects the anti-infective properties of the milk. If your baby is very small or not gaining weight, and you are pumping more than twice what he is being fed, pump the foremilk and freeze for later use then pump the hindmilk to take to the nursery. Human milk can be stored at room temperature for 4 hours, in the refrigerator for 4–8 days (put it in the freezer if it has not been used by then), in the freezer compartment of your refrigerator/freezer for 3 months, or in an upright or chest freezer for 3 months (Illustration 26).[75] Store in small quantities or single feeding portions to prevent waste.

HUMAN MILK STORAGE RECOMMENDATIONS FOR SICK OR PREMATURE BABIES*

Human Milk	Room Temperature (25° C or 77° F)	Refrigerator (4° C or 39° F)	Refrigerator/Freezer (-5° C or 5° F)	Freezer (-20° C or -4° F)
Fresh	4 hours	4-8 days	3 months	3 months
Thawed in refrigerator	Use within 1 hour or refrigerate	24 hours	Do not refreeze	Do not refreeze
Thawed in pan of warm water	Use right away	Do not save	Do not refreeze	Do not refreeze
Left in feeding container after feeding	Do not save	Do not save	Do not refreeze	Do not refreeze

Fresh breastmilk is best for your baby. Storage recommendations may vary with your baby's age and health.

GETTING TO KNOW YOUR BABY AS HIS CONDITION IMPROVES

As soon as your baby is stable and can be held for a period of time each day, ask his nurse if you can place him underneath your clothing and cuddle him skin-to-skin against your chest (kangaroo care). This early contact gives mothers and fathers a chance to care for their baby and to gain confidence in their ability to parent. Safe and secure against your chest, your body provides all the warmth your baby needs as he gets to know you. Plan to hold him like this for about an hour at a time. The most stressful time for the baby is when he is being taken out or put in the isolette, not the time he spends sleeping on your chest.

Both mothers and fathers can provide kangaroo care. Babies who are held skin-to-skin gain weight faster, move into an open crib sooner, and go home earlier.[76] Also, mothers who provide kangaroo care often breastfeed for longer periods of time. You may notice that your breasts leak while you are holding your baby skin-to-skin and that you are able to pump more milk after providing kangaroo care.

BEGINNING TO BREASTFEED A SICK OR PREMATURE BABY

Discuss your baby's readiness to breastfeed with the medical staff. Recent studies suggest that a baby's ability to suck, swallow, and breathe in an organized manner is the best indication of readiness to breastfeed and may appear as soon as 32 weeks gestation. Many babies can breast-feed, without showing signs of stress, days or weeks before they can bottle-feed.[77]

Once your baby is ready to breastfeed, ask for (or bring from home) a pillow to support your baby at your breast. The football hold or cross-cradle hold usually works best in the beginning (Illustration 16). Loosen his blanket so his arms can hug your breast. Support his back and shoulders (not his head) in the palm of your hand. His ear, shoulder, and hip should be in a straight line so his jaw can relax to open. Express a few drops of breastmilk onto your nipple and areola.

Support your breast with your other hand and shape the areola and nipple into a wedge. Gently touch his lips with your nipple. As he opens his mouth, continue holding your breast as you hug him to the breast. Resist the urge to press on his head, because that will make it difficult for him to swallow and breathe. The dancer's hand support is helpful for tiny babies with weak muscles. Using your thumb and first finger to

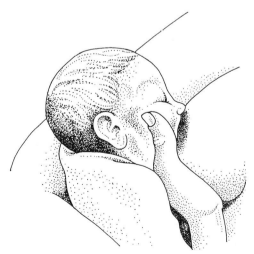

Illustration 27
The ***dancer's hand*** position can be helpful for tiny babies with weak muscles.

form a U-shape, support your baby's chin on the breast with your hand (Illustration 27).

If your milk is flowing freely, he may just lick and swallow. If your milk flows more slowly, he will start to suck and swallow. He should suck in bursts of at least 6 suck/swallows (some babies do many more) and then will pause before he sucks again. As he slows down, you can massage the breast to move more hindmilk into his mouth (Illustration 20).[78] Remember that he has never had to eat before — the milk was just dripped into his stomach, so he may not be really eager right away. These first breastfeedings are a learning experience for both of you, so relax and enjoy each moment. If you do not hear him swallow and your breast does not soften, his nurse can give him your breastmilk through a feeding tube (gavage feeding).

Often a mother is making more milk than her baby can take at first. If you are pumping 2–3 ounces per pumping session and your baby is only being fed 1 ounce per feeding, expect that he will only soften one breast. You will need to pump when you finish holding him. You may find that after your baby has breastfed you can pump more milk than usual for that time of day because you may get a stronger let-down when your baby breastfeeds than when you pump. Continue to pump after each feeding to soften your breasts until your baby is fully breast-feeding. If you are pumping more than twice what your baby is taking per feeding, pump one breast partially and then breastfeed on that breast. This will assure that your baby is getting the higher calorie hind-milk, which will help him to grow faster.

At first most premature babies will only be able to nipple (feed by mouth) once every 24 hours. The rest of the feedings will still be through a tube while the baby sleeps. Soon he will be ready for 2 breastfeedings a day, usually separated by at least 1–2 tube feedings. When he is ready for a third breastfeeding each day, you will want to talk to the medical staff about doing 2 breastfeedings in a row to save you time and to see if he has the energy to feed at the breast twice in a row. As he gets closer to coming home, he may start to gag on the feed-ing tube, which is a sign that he is maturing. A feeding tube can be put through his nose and left there between feedings, the nurse can cup feed him, or he can be bottle-fed (once he is breastfeeding easily, a bottle should not confuse him).

TIMING OF FEEDINGS

Premature babies go through several feeding patterns as they approach full term. If your baby is very small, he may start out with a continuous drip of milk into his stomach. Gradually the feedings will change to what is called a "bolus feeding," where a quantity of milk is given every 3 hours — the same pattern as a breastfeeding baby. Then, often at about 34–35 weeks gestation, babies seem to be able to eat more at one time, but awaken less frequently. If it is very difficult to wake your baby for feedings every 3 hours, talk with his doctor or nurse about moving him to a 4 hour schedule for a while. Expect that when he comes home he will change back to a 3 hour schedule as he gets closer to his due date. That is another sign that he is maturing. Since he is staying awake longer and getting more active, he needs to eat more often.

PROVIDING A SUPPLEMENT/SUBSTITUTE

Your milk supply may be low despite regular pumping, and breastmilk (your frozen milk or banked donor milk) or formula supplements may be necessary. To avoid nipple confusion caused by following each breast-feeding with a bottle-feeding, supplements can be given with a supplemental feeding device while you are breastfeeding[79] (Illustration 28).

A supplemental feeding device is a plastic container filled with human milk or formula that hangs on a cord around the mother's neck. A thin piece of plastic tubing stretches from the top of the container to the nipple of each breast, where the tubing is taped into place. When the baby breastfeeds, he receives milk from the breast and supplement from the container. Once the baby is breastfeeding well and a good milk supply is established, the supplement can be discontinued. To ease your mind, you can weigh your baby before and after feedings using a special baby scale. If breastmilk production remains low, talk with a lactation consultant, your doctor, or your baby's nurse about medication that can be prescribed to help increase your milk supply.[80]

As the condition of your baby improves and your confidence in your ability to care for your baby grows, you will be glad you chose to breastfeed. While breastfeeding a healthy, full term infant can be a challenge, breastfeeding a premature baby can be overwhelming at times. However, the bigger the challenge, the greater the rewards!

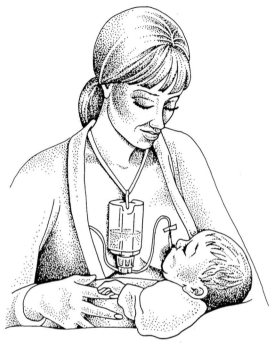

Illustration 28
You can supplement a baby at the breast using a supplemental feeding device.
(Example shown is a Supplemental Nursing System™ by Medela®.)

Breastfeeding Multiples

You can produce enough milk to totally meet the nutritional needs of two (or more) babies. The amount of milk you make depends on the amount removed from your breasts during breastfeedings or through milk expression. Early, frequent breastfeedings or milk expression, if one or more babies need special care, will help you get off to the best possible start. All the advantages of breastfeeding for mother and babies are multiplied when you give birth to two or more babies. Babies benefit from the perfect blend of nutrients and anti-infective properties that breastmilk provides. Mother benefits from the release of oxytocin that limits uterine bleeding, which can be greater after a multiple birth. Mother will appreciate the fact that breastfeeding requires little or no preparation, and Dad will value the cost savings. All will benefit from the enforced skin-to-skin contact that can help you get to know each baby as an individual.

PLANNING AHEAD

Be prepared to begin breastfeeding under many different circumstances. Surgical (cesarean) birth, preterm delivery, and other conditions resulting in a need for special care for one or more babies are more common with multiple births.

- Attend childbirth preparation and surgical birth classes early in pregnancy, beginning in your fourth or fifth month.

- Share and discuss information about breastfeeding multiples with your partner, family, and friends.

- Locate resources for buying or renting a breast pump, should milk expression be necessary.

- Contact breastfeeding and parents of multiples support groups, such as La Leche League and a Mothers of Twins club. Ask if someone can put you in touch with another mother who is breastfeeding or has successfully breastfed the same number of multiples.

- Choose a pediatrician, family practice physician, or pediatric nurse practitioner who is knowledgeable about breastfeeding and who has cared for other sets of successfully breastfed multiples.

- Ask your partner, a family member, or friend to stay with you at night while you are in the hospital, so you will have extra help when you begin to breastfeed your babies.

- Arrange for daily or round-the-clock household help for several weeks after the babies come home from the hospital.

- Set a goal to continue breastfeeding for at least 6–8 weeks after birth, no matter how difficult it may seem at times.

The encouragement and support of those close to you, another breast-feeding mother of multiples, and your babies' pediatric care provider will give you confidence in your ability to produce all that your babies need.

BEGINNING TO BREASTFEED

Healthy, full term multiples. Ideally, your babies' first breastfeeding will occur soon after birth. Healthy newborns who are born at, or close to, full term usually search for and crawl to their mother's breast within an hour of birth.[81] Although rooming-in, or a modified version of it, is possible with twins, you may need the help of a family member or friend if you have a surgical delivery or triplets. It is easier to breastfeed frequently when babies are accessible, and your confidence in handling them can grow when a nurse or a lactation consultant is available.

When rooming-in is not possible, ask that all babies be brought to you for all feedings. Each multiple is a single baby, needing 8–12 breastfeedings in a 24-hour period. In the beginning, it may seem confusing if each baby has a somewhat different, albeit normal, breastfeeding pattern. Until you have a better sense of each baby's breastfeeding style, it may help to write down feedings and wet and dirty diapers on a checklist that is color-coded for each multiple.

Preterm or sick newborn multiples. When multiples' conditions require a stay in a newborn intensive care unit (NICU), you will want to begin expressing your milk within hours of giving birth if your condition permits. If you are sick and unable to express milk on your own, a nurse, lactation consultant, family member, or friend can help you use a breast pump. You should express milk as often as you would breastfeed your babies. Do not worry about the quantity of milk you express. The goal of early, frequent milk expression is to let your body know that a lot of milk will be needed in a few days. The sooner and more often you express your breasts, the sooner you will produce greater amounts of milk.

Most mothers find it easier to manage frequent milk expression when they use an electric self-cycling breast pump. When a double collection kit is attached, it is possible to pump both breasts at once (Illustration 24). This saves time and appears to benefit milk production.[82] Establishing a routine, pumping at about the same times each day, usually produces greater amounts of expressed breastmilk.

Begin by pumping at least 8 times a day. To increase milk production for multiples, increase the number of pumping sessions as babies' conditions improve or any time you notice a decline in breastmilk volume. (Many mothers notice variations in milk production when pumping for preterm or sick babies.) By the time the babies go to breast, you will want to be pumping about 8–12 times in 24 hours (see "Breastfeeding the Premature Baby," p. 83).

Sometimes one (or more) of the babies is able to room in with you. Or one may be discharged earlier, while the other(s) must remain in the NICU. In this situation, breastfeed each baby that is with you 8–12 times in 24 hours. You can pump for any multiple(s) in the NICU. To save time, pump one breast while one baby breastfeeds on the other breast. If you don't think you are ready to coordinate pumping while breastfeeding, pump both breasts immediately after a breastfeeding, or pump between breastfeedings.

Newborn feeding difficulties. Multiples, including those born at or close to full term, are more likely to be affected by pregnancy, labor, and delivery situations that can influence their initial ability to latch on and breastfeed correctly. One multiple may be affected more than the other(s). In addition, some preterm or sick multiples have difficulty making the transition to the breast because of exposure to other feeding methods that interfere with oral behaviors needed for effective breast-feeding.

These types of feeding difficulties may last from several hours to several weeks, but they tend to be short-lived. Most can be resolved with patience and persistence. However, "short-lived" may seem like forever when you are sleep deprived and juggling breastfeedings, supplementary feedings, and breast pumping sessions! Contact a breastfeeding moth-ers' support group and/or an IBCLC certified lactation consultant to help you. They can offer practical problem-solving strategies and pro-vide moral support.

DEVELOPING A FEEDING ROUTINE

Almost any method of coordinating breastfeedings will work as long as each baby breastfeeds 8–12 times in 24 hours. Some mothers breastfeed each baby on both breasts at every feeding. However, many mothers find it less confusing to feed one baby only on one breast at each feeding. This also makes it possible to breastfeed two babies at the same time. If you let each baby breastfeed as long as desired, so that the baby, not the mother, chooses when to end a feeding, your milk supply will quickly increase to meet your babies' needs.

To stimulate milk production equally in both breasts, it is a good idea to alternate babies and breasts. You may alternate babies and breasts for each feeding, but many mothers find it is easier to alternate babies and breasts on a daily basis. For example, today Baby A (and Baby C) feeds on the right breast and Baby B (and Baby D) on the left. Then tomorrow Baby A (and Baby C) feeds on the left breast and Baby B (and Baby D) on the right. Mothers of odd-numbered multiples may have to alternate babies and breasts more often than every 24 hours. If you feed the baby who wakes first, you probably will find that the one(s) feeding second on a breast and last will be the one(s) ready to eat first at the next feeding.

Some mothers assign babies a specific breast. Milk production in each breast then adapts to that individual baby's needs. However, you may find yourself with breasts of very different sizes! Also, you may find another multiple unwilling to breastfeed on the unfamiliar side if a situation arises in which one baby cannot breastfeed for any period of time, such as during a nursing strike (see "What are nursing strikes?" p. 142), which are more common with multiples than with single-birth infants. If you choose to have each baby always feed at a specific breast, vary feeding positions from feeding to feeding.

Simultaneous feedings. Breastfeeding simultaneously (two babies at once) can save a lot of time. Some mothers always breastfeed two; others never breastfeed simultaneously. Most mothers do both. They simultaneously feed two for some feedings and feed the babies separately for others. It usually depends on the babies' and mothers' needs during any given feeding.

Don't begin simultaneous feedings until you feel comfortable positioning and helping a single baby latch on to the breast. At least one baby should be able to latch on and breastfeed without difficulty before you attempt to feed two at once. If both infants demonstrate any incorrect breastfeeding behaviors, simultaneous feedings may reinforce those behaviors.

Even if you or the babies find simultaneous feeding difficult to master in the early weeks, keep trying. It usually becomes much easier after several weeks or a few months when babies have become skilled at latching on to the breast. Use pillows to hold the babies in position, so your hands are free to help with latch-on. Many mothers prefer the support of a firm breastfeeding pillow. You may want to work with pillows already available in your home before purchasing a special pillow, since some mothers find that pillows with a little "give" are more useful for positioning babies.

The following positions are the ones used most often for simultaneous breastfeedings (Illustration 29):

Double Football/Double Clutch Hold. In this position, a baby's body is tucked under each of your arms (or is supported on a pillow at your side) while a baby's head is supported in each of your hands (or on a pillow). A mother's hands are free to help babies latch on when pillows are used to hold babies in place, so many mothers learn this position first. This position also limits pressure on the incision area after a surgical birth. However, it can be the least "hands-on" position, which is a disadvantage.

Criss-Cross/Double Cradle Hold. With a baby's head cradled in the bend of each arm and the babies' chests rolled to face your chest, criss-cross the babies' bodies in front of your abdomen. A pillow on your lap and under each elbow often adds comfort and support. You may be more comfortable if you place your feet on a stool, sit in a recliner, or tailor-sit (Indian-style) on the floor. This position increases skin-to-skin contact between mother and each baby and enhances baby-to-baby contact.

Some mothers adjust this position with older babies by cradling each baby's head and supporting a baby's body parallel to each of mother's

Illustration 29
Breastfeeding multiples simultaneously
saves time and energy.

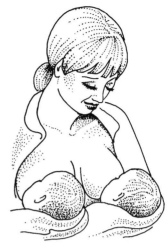

**COMBINATION CRADLE-FOOTBALL/
LAYERED/PARALLEL HOLDS**

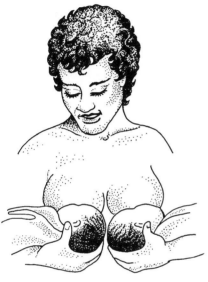

DOUBLE FOOTBALL/DOUBLE CLUTCH HOLD

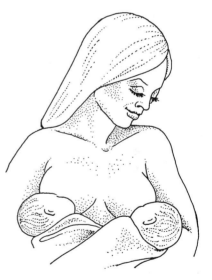

CRISS-CROSS/DOUBLE CRADLE HOLD

legs. To breastfeed in bed, a mother can lie on her back, and, with a baby's head cradled in each arm, lay a baby's body along each arm, parallel to each side of her abdomen. The babies' heads and bodies are rolled toward and face each breast.

Combination Cradle-Football/Layered/Parallel Holds. With Baby A held in the traditional cradle hold, Baby B's head is supported in your hand or on a pillow or "layered" gently on Baby A's abdomen. Tuck Baby B's body under your arm or lay his body on a pillow out to the side at a right angle from your body. This position lends itself better to discreet breastfeeding. It is a "hands-on" position, yet one or both hands can be free to help assist with latch-on.

PARTIAL BREASTFEEDING

Full or nearly full breastfeeding is ideal for babies, but it may not always be possible with multiples. Partial breastfeeding provides babies with varying degrees of nutritional and anti-infective benefits. The benefits depend on the number of breastfeedings (or amount of breastmilk) each receives. Regardless of the amount of breastmilk received, research indicates that any amount of breastfeeding, or breastmilk, is much better than none.

Mothers choose partial breastfeeding for a variety of reasons. Sometimes they want some relief with feedings. Often partial breastfeeding is chosen because of ongoing feeding difficulties. Others choose partial breastfeeding when they return to work outside the home. Some mothers partially breastfeed, but babies still receive only their mother's milk. These mothers pump their breasts once or twice a day, and their babies then receive the expressed milk from a bottle or cup.

Because breastfeeding means more than good nutrition for babies and mothers, fully breastfeeding one (or more) and fully bottle-feeding the other(s) should be avoided if at all possible. It may lead to long-lasting differences in a mother's feelings for her babies. In the rare instances when it is necessary, mothers should be aware of the concerns and increase skin-to-skin contact with any bottle-fed baby.

Plans compatible with breastfeeding. Partial breastfeeding is more successful when bottles are offered on a limited basis. To maintain adequate milk production and avoid unanticipated weaning, breastfeed at least 8–12 times a day. For example, you would breastfeed each twin at least 4–6 times in 24 hours, each triplet at least 3–4 times, and each quadruplet at least 2–3 times.

Most mothers choose to offer a bottle during the night or in the evening when babies tend to cluster-feed. You can breastfeed first, then ask Dad to offer each baby a bottle to complement or "top off" an evening feeding. Other options include Dad bottle-feeding one (or more) while you breastfeed the other(s), or Dad bottle-feeding all babies during one night feeding while you breastfeed all during the next feeding.

Employment. Employed mothers of multiples usually find it is easier to continue breastfeeding when they rent or purchase a portable electric self-cycling breast pump that can be used with a double collection kit. If you already have a double collection kit, you will save money by renting a compatible brand of pump. Establishing a pumping routine is especially important for a mother pumping for multiples. Try to pump every 2–3 hours while away from the babies. If you want your babies to receive only your breastmilk for their first few months, you may have to schedule 1 or 2 additional 10–15 minute pumping sessions each day to maintain adequate milk production.

Breastmilk feeding. Mothers sometimes choose to exclusively bottle-feed expressed breastmilk when one or more babies experiences an ongoing difficulty at the breast. Short-term breastmilk feeding can give a mother a chance to focus on increasing or maintaining milk production when breast pumping, breastfeedings, and supplementary feedings have become overwhelming. There are mothers who breastmilk feed for longer periods. Some choose to continue pumping 8–12 times a day for many months and offer the expressed milk in a bottle or cup.

PERSPECTIVE

Each of your multiple babies has the same needs as any single-birth infant, so multiples require more time and effort no matter how they are fed. Remembering this may help on those days when you feel as if you have competed in a breastfeeding marathon and just "hit the wall." When you wonder if you will ever experience the "joys" of breastfeeding, it can help to recall that your babies have been enjoying the benefits of breastfeeding and breastmilk from day 1.

Your multiples will be breastfeeding babies for only a brief period of time. Maintain perspective by accepting all offers of help, surrounding yourself with a supportive network of family and friends, and finding the humor amid the chaos! Confidence in your body's ability to make enough milk, and in your babies' ability to get all they need through breastfeeding, will grow as your babies grow. Before you know it, you will be numbering yourself among the many mothers who have successfully breastfed multiples.

Breastfeeding the Baby with Jaundice

Jaundice in the newborn is a common, complex, and poorly understood problem. As a result, management of the breastfed baby with jaundice often causes confusion and concern for parents.[83] Jaundice occurs in at least 50% of full term infants and 75% of premature infants. Your baby's skin and the whites of his eyes look yellow. In addition, your baby may be sleepy and feed poorly.

Jaundice occurs when there is too much bilirubin in the blood. Bilirubin is a substance found in red blood cells. During pregnancy, babies need extra red blood cells to meet their oxygen needs. After birth, these red blood cells break down, and bilirubin is released into the blood. The baby's liver removes the bilirubin from the blood and transfers it to the lower bowel where it is expelled in the stool. Because newborn babies' livers are immature, it is hard for them to remove the large amount of bilirubin that collects after birth. In addition, when rules or routines limit the number of breastfeedings, a baby has fewer stools, and the bilirubin is reabsorbed into the blood.

Physiologic jaundice. Physiologic jaundice usually occurs 3 days after birth and disappears within 10–12 days. Recent studies found no difference in the peak level of bilirubin between breast and bottle-fed babies; however, breastfeeding may cause bilirubin levels to remain elevated for longer periods of time.[84] While many doctors question the need to treat breastfed babies with physiologic jaundice, other doctors recommend water or formula supplementation, phototherapy (placing the baby in indirect sunlight), or stopping breastfeeding for a brief period of time.[85] Discuss the choices carefully with your baby's doctor in an effort to avoid unnecessary confusion.

Pathologic jaundice. Pathologic jaundice is caused by blood incompatibility or liver disease. Different from physiologic jaundice, pathologic jaundice occurs within 24 hours after birth, and the bilirubin level may rise quickly. Prompt medical attention is necessary.

Breastmilk jaundice. Breastmilk jaundice can occur in 30% of all breast-fed newborns. The cause of breastmilk jaundice is unclear. There may be a substance in the milk of some women that affects liver function. Breastmilk jaundice appears 4–6 days after birth. Bilirubin levels peak 10–14 days after birth and can remain elevated for several weeks or several months. In rare cases, if the bilirubin level continues to rise after day 14, your baby's doctor may suggest that you rotate breastmilk and formula feedings for 24 hours or stop breastfeeding for 24 hours and pump or hand express. Because each of these options might interfere with continued breastfeeding, discuss them fully with your baby's doctor.

Breastfeeding jaundice. Breastmilk jaundice should not be confused with breastfeeding jaundice. Breastfeeding jaundice occurs when babies are not breastfed often enough. Expect to breastfeed every 1–3 hours during the day and every 2–3 hours at night (8–12 breastfeedings in a 24 hour period). Fewer feedings result in fewer stools and an increase in the likelihood of jaundice.

Often it is easy to identify the cause of jaundice. Many times a medical examination is necessary. Jaundice that occurs after you leave the hospital should be reported to your baby's doctor.

TO PREVENT JAUNDICE:

- Breastfeed as soon as possible after birth. Colostrum is a natural laxative that causes bowel movements (stools). Early, frequent stools limit the reabsorption of bilirubin.

- Breastfeed at least 8–12 times in 24 hours. Frequent feedings result in frequent stools, which increase the passage of bilirubin and decrease the likelihood of jaundice. Expect at least 3 stools a day for the first 3 days and at least 4 stools a day for the next 4 weeks.[39, 40]

❧ Breastfeed well on the first breast before offering the second breast. This will produce high calorie, high fat feedings, which in turn will increase the number of stools and limit the reabsorption of bilirubin.

❧ Avoid water or formula supplements. As long as you have a good supply of colostrum or breastmilk and your baby is breastfeeding 8–12 times in 24 hours and passing 4–6 stools a day, continued breastfeeding is all your baby needs.[85]

JAUNDICE IN THE NEWBORN

TYPES OF JAUNDICE	SIGNS	BEGINS
PHYSIOLOGIC JAUNDICE Affects 50–75% of newborns	❧ Skin and whites of the eyes look yellow	3 days after birth
PATHOLOGIC JAUNDICE Very rare	❧ Skin and whites of the eyes look yellow ❧ Baby may be sleepy and feed poorly	Within 24 hours of birth
BREASTMILK JAUNDICE Affects 30% of breastfed newborns	❧ Skin and whites of the eyes look yellow ❧ Baby is: • alert and active • breastfeeding at least 8 times a day • gaining weight • passing at least 4 stools a day	5–7 days after birth
BREASTFEEDING JAUNDICE Frequency varies widely	❧ Skin and whites of the eyes look yellow ❧ Baby is: • sleepy • breastfeeding fewer than 8 times a day • losing weight • passing fewer than 4 stools a day	3–5 days after birth

TO TREAT JAUNDICE

❧ Sometimes babies with jaundice are treated with phototherapy (light treatment) using a fluorescent and/or fiberoptic light. When a baby is exposed to the light source, his bilirubin level goes down. If an overhead light source is used, a small mask may be placed over the baby's eyes. Phototherapy will increase your baby's fluid needs, so remember to breastfeed frequently, every 1–3 hours. Babies with jaundice, especially those receiving phototherapy, may be sleepy, so you will need to work at waking them to feed. (see "Suggestions for Waking a Sleepy Baby," p. 50).

❧ You can place your baby outdoors in indirect sunlight for brief periods of time if the weather permits. However, be careful to avoid sunburn.

Lasts	Cause(s)	Treatment
10–12 days	❧ Breakdown of excess red blood cells ❧ Immature newborn liver	❧ Breastfeed at least 8–12 times a day ❧ Check bilirubin level as needed ❧ Place baby in indirect sunlight for brief periods; avoid sunburn
Bilirubin level rises quickly and continues to rise until medical treatment is started	❧ Blood incompatibility (ABO, Rh) ❧ Liver disease	❧ Medical evaluation ❧ Breastfeed at least 8–12 times a day ❧ Phototherapy ❧ Blood transfusion
Bilirubin level usually peaks 10–14 days after birth but can remain elevated for 16 weeks	❧ Unknown; may be something in the mother's milk	❧ Breastfeed at least 8–12 times a day ❧ Check bilirubin level regularly ❧ If level continues to rise after 14 days: • phototherapy • rotate breastfeedings and formula feedings • interrupt breastfeeding for 24 hours
Bilirubin level usually peaks 3–5 days after birth but may continue to rise if baby is breastfeeding poorly	❧ Fewer than 8 breastfeedings a day ❧ Time limits for each feeding (mother-led) ❧ Poor breastmilk production, release, and/or transfer	❧ Breastfeed at least 8–12 times a day ❧ Breastfeed as long as the baby wishes (baby-led feeding) ❧ Look for signs of milk production, milk release, and milk transfer ❧ Supplement, if necessary, with breastmilk or formula

Breastfeeding the Baby
with a Family History of Allergic Disease

Parents who have a personal or family history of allergic disease such as asthma, hay fever, allergic rhinitis, chronic ear infections, or eczema should seriously consider breastfeeding their babies. This is particularly important if both parents suffer from allergic disease or have a previous child with allergic problems.[86]

Human milk feeding for at least the first year of life can reduce the incidence of allergic symptoms (gas, diarrhea, vomiting, fussiness, and skin rashes) and the development of food sensitivity and upper respiratory infections in sensitive babies.[19] Early introduction of foods other than human milk greatly increases the potential for developing food allergies.[20] Human milk alone is recommended for the first six months, avoiding all formula and solid food supplements.

When supplements are introduced, the new foods should be added one at a time at weekly intervals. This will let you clearly identify those foods that produce allergic symptoms. Cow's milk, eggs, peanuts, peanut butter, and wheat should be completely avoided during the first year of life. After the first year, cow's milk and wheat can be added, but eggs should be avoided until 18 months of age and peanuts and peanut butter avoided until 3 years of age. This will not eliminate the development of sensitivity to these foods but will greatly reduce the likelihood of sensitivity. If formula supplements are necessary, avoid cow's milk-based formulas and choose soy-based formulas instead. For extremely sensitive babies or if severe symptoms occur and breastfeeding is not possible or human milk is not available, a hypo-allergenic formula can be suggested by your baby's doctor.

Occasionally allergic symptoms develop in exclusively breastfed babies. Food proteins can be found in human milk in small quantities. For extremely sensitive babies, these proteins may occur in large enough amounts to cause allergic symptoms. In an effort to identify the cause of the symptoms, the mother's diet will need to be restricted. Foods eaten by the mother that most often cause reactions in the baby are cow's milk, eggs, nuts, and wheat (Illustration 30). You will need to eliminate

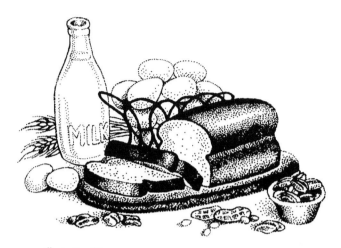

Illustration 30
Foods eaten by the mother that may cause allergic symptoms
in her baby include cow's milk, eggs, nuts, and wheat.

these foods from your diet for 3 weeks, then re-introduce the foods one at a time, leaving 5–7 days between. It is unlikely that all the foods are the cause of the symptoms. By re-introducing the foods one at a time, it should be possible to determine the food (or foods) that is the cause. If the restricted diet does not improve the baby's symptoms, the mother's diet can be returned to normal immediately, and the baby's doctor should be consulted. If the baby's symptoms are severe, a board certified allergist should be consulted before the foods are re-introduced.

The following suggestions will complement the use of human milk in achieving the goal of fewer symptoms in allergic children.[87]

- Reduce dust and dust mite exposure in the home. Cover your mattresses with special dust mite preventive covers, limit the use of wall-to-wall carpeting throughout the house, and change furnace filters frequently.

- Avoid furry and feathered animals during the first 5 years of a child's life. It is much easier to refuse a pet than to get rid of a pet that has become part of the family.

❧ Keep babies and children in a smoke-free environment. This includes the homes of friends and relatives as well as automobiles. Early and chronic exposure to smoke is associated with an increased incidence of respiratory illnesses and early onset of asthma.

❧ Avoid child care settings, nursery school environments, and church nurseries. Heavy and early exposure to viral infections can cause chronic diseases such as ear infections and infectious asthma. Early and frequent viral diseases can cause a significant increase in allergic antibodies. If child care outside the home is necessary, choose a setting with fewer children to reduce the potential for problems.

Breastfeeding, environmental controls, animal avoidance, smoke avoidance, and dietary management do not prevent allergic disease. However, in many cases, they will delay the onset of symptoms for many years and limit the severity of symptoms when they do occur. This will allow the baby to mature and be better able to handle those symptoms that may develop.

Science has shown time and again that breastfed babies, both allergic and non-allergic, have fewer acute infections, have less risk of chronic disease, and respond better to immunizations. Human milk is truly the food of choice for every baby and child.

Breastfeeding
and the Working Mother

Many mothers who work outside the home continue to breastfeed. It takes a little extra planning and preparation to combine working and breastfeeding, but the benefits are worth it (see "Benefits of Breastfeeding," p. 17).

- Breastfeeding keeps a mother and baby close even when they are apart.

- Breastmilk keeps a baby healthy (especially those in group child care centers).

- Mothers of healthy babies miss less work, lose less income, and have less worry from sick babies.

- Breastfeeding saves money; mothers who breastfeed do not have to spend their earnings on large amounts of infant formula or foods to replace their breastmilk.

Many mothers do not realize how easy it is to combine breastfeeding and working, so they stop breastfeeding when they return to work. However, as the number of working mothers increases, employers are becoming more supportive of breastfeeding. In the past, few employers considered breastfeeding beneficial, but today many see how breast-feeding can help their business. Breastfeeding and working can be a win-win-win situation for mother, baby, and employer.

KEY POINTS TO THINK ABOUT

How do you plan to feed your baby when you return to work?

How will you express your milk or feed your baby during work hours?

How will you complete your work duties and take care of your breastfeeding needs?

How will you combine work duties and household chores?

START PLANNING WHILE YOU ARE PREGNANT

Let your employer know as soon as possible that you are pregnant. Use this time to learn about the company's maternity policies, benefits, and work options. Discuss these options with your employer; suggest new options if necessary.

- How long is your maternity leave? Is it paid or unpaid? How much leave can you take without losing your job or position? Does your national, state, or local government have a family medical leave law? (Some laws provide up to 12 weeks of maternity leave.)

- How many hours per week will you be expected to work when you return?

- Does your company offer work options such as flex-time (adjusting when you start and stop each work day), job-sharing (sharing a full-time job with another person), part-time work, compressed work week (fewer days with longer hours), or telecommuting (working from home)?

- Does company policy allow you to leave the work site during the day or have a baby at work part- or full-time?

- Does your company offer onsite child care? If not, is this an option the company might consider?

- Does your company have a policy on breastfeeding or breastmilk expression at the work site? Does your company provide breast pumps or breastfeeding rooms? Does your company give employees time and support to breastfeed or express milk during the work day? (This is most important.)

DECIDE WHEN YOU WILL RETURN TO WORK

Once you know the policies of your company, you can think about your options. The longer you and your baby can be together, the more stable your milk supply will be. Also, the older the baby is when you return to work, the less you may need to pump during the work day. It is best to take as much time off as possible. Whether you return to work after 6 weeks, 6 months, or 6 years will depend on your own needs and circumstances. For many mothers the decision to return to work is not a choice but a necessity. Mothers with limited sources of income and no paid maternity leave have to return to paid work as soon as possible.

DECIDE HOW MANY HOURS A WEEK YOU WOULD LIKE TO WORK AND WHEN

Those mothers able to return to work part-time, at first, find it easier to work and breastfeed. A part-time schedule gives you a chance to rest and care for yourself and your baby, and makes the return to work easier. Some mothers who return to work full-time right away are able to adjust their schedules with flexible work hours that allow extra time during the work day for expressing milk or breastfeeding. Others compress their work week, working full-time in fewer than 5 days; for example, working a 40-hour week as 4 10-hour days or 3 13-hour days.

DECIDE WHERE AND WHEN YOU CAN EXPRESS OR BREASTFEED DURING WORK HOURS

If you plan to return to work shortly after your baby is born and want to express or breastfeed at the work site, think about where and when this can happen. You won't know how long breastfeeding or expressing your milk will take until after your baby is born and you have a chance to practice. If you plan to use a breast pump, find out if your employer provides pumps or supplies or ask for one as a baby gift. Look for places at the work site where you can express your milk or breastfeed such as a private office, a health clinic, or a child care center. You may need to be creative as you look for space, privacy, and comfort.

DECIDE WHO WILL TAKE CARE OF YOUR BABY DURING WORK HOURS

Choosing child care is an important task. While cost and convenience are necessary considerations, choosing someone you trust who understands and supports breastfeeding is most important. Child care options include taking the baby with you to work, leaving the baby with an individual, either in your home or their home, taking the baby to a child care center, or arranging work schedules so that one parent is always available to care for the baby. If you plan to breastfeed your baby during work hours, you might want to choose an individual or child care center near your work place or arrange to have the baby brought to you for feedings. When you are interviewing different child care providers, ask them about their policies concerning breastfed babies (see "Choosing a Child Care Provider," p. 112). You need to know that your baby is getting the care you want. If you have a child care center at your work site, let your employer know how much you value this employee benefit. If you do not have onsite child care, get information from other companies who provide this service and share the information with your employer.

CHOOSING A CHILD CARE PROVIDER

When looking for a child care provider, begin by choosing someone who understands and supports breastfeeding and who is licensed or certified (especially if you are considering a group child care center). Take plenty of time to interview possible providers and make at least one unplanned visit.

Choose a provider who:

- provides a safe, clean place for your baby.

- encourages you to breastfeed onsite when you drop off or pick up your baby, as well as during the day.

- has trained staff who have experience with infant care and will help meet your baby's special needs.

- is near your work site, if you are able to leave work to feed your baby.

- knows how to safely handle your expressed breastmilk and feed your baby.

GET SUPPORT FROM YOUR EMPLOYER, SUPERVISOR, AND CO-WORKERS

Before you begin your maternity leave, discuss your ideas with your supervisor and co-workers. Encourage them to support your efforts to breastfeed after your return to work. See if you can get them to commit their support in writing. Some ideas for building and maintaining support with your employer include:

❧ Talking to other working, breastfeeding mothers about their situations at their work sites. If they have had positive experiences, see if their supervisors would be willing to discuss the arrangement(s) with your employer. Sometimes employers are more willing to follow where others have already shown success, rather than blazing the trail themselves.

❧ Sharing research data or publications on how your breastfeeding can help their business. For instance, breastfed babies are typically sick fewer times, even when placed in group day care centers. Less sickness on the baby's part means less absence on your part, which means better productivity for the company. One study found that non-breastfeeding mothers were absent from the work site 3 times more often (due to babies' illnesses) than breastfeeding mothers.[14]

❧ Investigating ways to meet your job responsibilities while you are expressing/feeding, so that your employer, supervisor, and co-workers will agree that you are doing your fair share of the work.

TAKE CARE OF YOURSELF AND YOUR BABY DURING YOUR BIRTH AND MATERNITY LEAVE

Enjoy this precious time with your baby to the fullest. Breastfeed early and often to help your baby learn good breastfeeding practices and to establish a good milk supply. Avoid pacifiers, bottles, or foods other than breastmilk for the first 4 weeks after birth. These can confuse your baby's sucking pattern and decrease your milk supply.

LEARN HOW TO EXPRESS AND COLLECT YOUR BREASTMILK

If you plan to give your baby breastmilk during your work day, you will need to learn how to express and collect. You can practice hand expression as soon as your milk supply increases, 5–7 days after birth. About 3 weeks after birth, you can begin to use a simple hand pump, a battery-operated pump, or an electric pump (see "Suggestions for Choosing a Breast Pump," p. 127). Practice early and often so that you will have time to learn this important skill before you return to work. Your first attempts at milk expression may produce only enough milk to cover the bottom of the collection container. Don't get discouraged. Much like the art of breastfeeding, success comes with practice (see "Collection and Storage of Breastmilk," p. 121).

After you have expressed your milk, you can store it in just about any food-safe container. There are even some plastic bags made just for breastmilk. Use something that is not likely to break, tear, or tip over in the refrigerator or freezer.

If you are expressing early on, and your baby is breastfeeding well, freeze your milk for later use. Label it with the date it was expressed. Breastmilk can be stored at room temperature for 4–8 hours, in the refrigerator for 4–8 days, in the freezer section of your refrigerator/freezer for 3 months, and in a upright or chest freezer for 6 months.[74]

As your baby gets older and your return to work gets closer, store your milk in single servings. Of course, your baby may want a bit more or less than this amount on any given day. If your baby seems hungrier than usual, feel free to make up larger servings for your baby's child care provider, or send along extra servings. Remember to adjust serving size as your baby grows.

ESTIMATE THE SIZE OF A SINGLE SERVING DURING THE FIRST 3 MONTHS

Babies eat about 2½ ounces (oz.) each day for every pound (lb.) they weigh. For example, an 8 lb. baby would eat 2½ oz. x 8 lb. or 20 oz. a day. Divide this amount by the number of feedings and you can estimate the size of a single feeding. If this baby breastfeeds 10 times a day, 20 oz. ÷ 10 feedings = 2 oz. per feeding.

INTRODUCE A NEW FEEDING METHOD AND/OR A BREASTMILK SUBSTITUTE

Once your baby is breastfeeding well, about 4 weeks after birth, you can introduce a new feeding method. If you do this too soon you can confuse your baby's sucking pattern and decrease your milk supply. However, if your work schedule requires that you be away from your baby during feeding times, you need to know that he will accept food from something other than the breast and from someone other than you.

What to substitute
Depending on the baby's age and ability, you can use expressed breastmilk, infant formula, or solid food. Doctors recommend breastmilk alone for the first 6 months. If you cannot give just breastmilk, your baby's doctor can recommend an infant formula. After the first 6 months, solid foods can be slowly introduced, but breastmilk or infant formula should still be fed through the first year of life.

How to substitute
You can use a cup, medicine dropper, hollow-handled medicine spoon, or bottle, whichever you, your baby, and your child care provider prefer. Should you choose to place the substitute in a bottle, try different nipple shapes and sizes until you find one that the baby will accept. Let someone other than you offer the substitute — your baby expects meals from you to come from your breast, not a cup or a bottle! In fact, you may want to leave the room during the feeding — some babies refuse substitutes when the real thing is nearby. Father, grandmother, baby-sitter, brother, or sister may be more than happy to offer the feeding.

Some mothers and babies avoid substitutes by *reverse-cycle* breastfeeding. Reverse-cycle breastfeeding means letting the baby sleep during the day while you are at work and breastfeeding in the evening and at night when you are together.

DECIDE HOW YOU WILL COMBINE HOUSEHOLD CHORES AND WORK DUTIES

When both parents work full-time outside the home, household chores are often shared. While cooking, cleaning, doing laundry, paying bills, grocery shopping, and running errands take time and energy, now breastfeeding and child care must be added to the To Do List!

❧ Sit down with your partner and make a list of household chores.

❧ Decide which chores have to be done and which can be put off. Divide up the rest.

RETURN TO WORK

During your pregnancy and maternity leave, you laid out your plan. You and your baby have learned to breastfeed. Now it is time to put these plans into action (Illustration 31).

2 weeks before your scheduled return to work:

❧ Discuss your plans with your supervisor. Assure her/him that you will be able to maintain your milk supply along with your daily and weekly work schedule.

❧ See how much time you will need each work day to wake, dress, and feed yourself and your baby, and travel to child care and work.

❧ Let your baby-sitter and baby spend time together so they can get to know each other.

❧ Begin to establish a milk expression schedule, if you will be expressing milk at work.

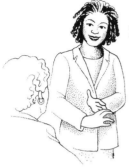

2nd trimester – Meet with your employer.

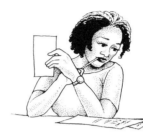

3rd trimester –
Choose child care;
attend a prenatal
breastfeeding class.

Birth – Breastfeed as soon as possible.

1–2 weeks – Breastfeed 8–12 times a day.

2–4 weeks – Learn to express and collect breastmilk; freeze milk for later use.

4–6 weeks – Introduce a breastmilk or formula substitute.

6–12 weeks – Delay your return to work for 12 weeks if possible.

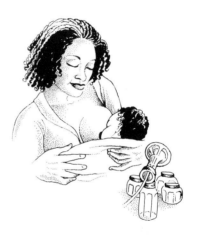

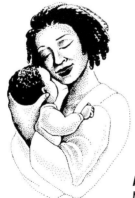

2 weeks prior to your return to work –
Decide how much time you will need each work day.

1 week prior to your return to work – Hold a dress rehearsal.

After you return to work –
Make the most of your time together.

Illustration 31
Many mothers combine breastfeeding and working. You simply need to plan ahead.

- If you will not be able to express milk at work, drop 1 feeding during the day and introduce a substitute so that your milk supply has a chance to adjust. Allow 3–5 days before dropping another breastfeeding, if needed.

- Introduce a substitute to your baby at the time you would otherwise breastfeed.

- Start making extra meals for you and your partner and storing them in the freezer.

1 week before your scheduled return to work:

- Continue your expression and breastfeeding schedule so that it will be close to what you will be doing when you return to work.

- Leave your baby with the baby-sitter for a few hours 2–3 times this week so they can get to know one another better.

- Hold a dress rehearsal of your new morning routine on 1–2 days this week and make changes as needed.

- Try to get plenty of sleep so that you are ready for your return to work.

When you return to work:

- Take it a day at a time. If work has piled up while you were away, relax and do your best to catch up.

- Breastfeed your baby right before you leave him with the sitter. This will limit the amount of milk you will need to express while you are apart.

- Express or breastfeed according to your established routine. You will probably need to make small adjustments depending on your work schedule. Try to pump or breastfeed a little early rather than a little late. Many times the hours rush by, and you may find yourself having gone longer than planned. Unfortunately, if you do not express or breastfeed, you will be uncomfortably full, your milk supply may decrease, and you will have a greater chance of leaking.

- Breastfeed your baby right after you return from work. If your breasts are very full or you have a long commute home, you may want to breastfeed before you leave the child care center. This will keep you and your baby happy. Ask your child care provider not to feed the baby for 1–2 hours before your planned return, so that he will be ready to eat when you get there.

- Breastfeed more often in the evenings and on weekends when you and your baby are together. This will help to maintain your milk supply.

- Talk to your supervisor about how things are going. Be positive and thankful, but also be realistic if there are difficulties.

- Take care of yourself — commit to getting enough sleep and eating a healthy diet.

- Give your baby at least one substitute feeding each day during any days off work (weekends, vacations, holidays).

Regardless of how well you prepare for your return to work, there will still be a period of adjustment. Excitement, nervousness, guilt, sadness, and joy are a few of the emotions you may experience. These feelings are normal. With time you will adjust priorities and establish routines, and your confidence in your decision will grow. Support and encouragement from people around you is important, so don't hesitate to ask for help.

Any amount of breastfeeding is wonderful. More important than how long you breastfeed or how often is that it be enjoyable for mother, father, and baby.

Collection and Storage of Human Milk

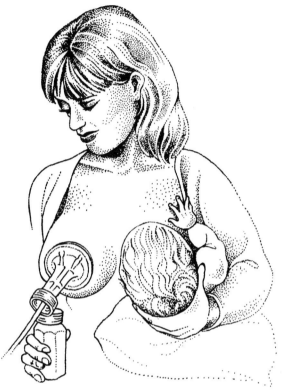

Illustration 32
Pumping one breast while the baby breastfeeds on the opposite breast
can increase the amount of milk expressed.

Breastmilk can be collected by hand expression, hand pump, battery-operated pump, or electric pump. Mothers who plan to pump now and then
will find that hand expression or a hand pump works well. Mothers who
need to pump daily or for many weeks or months may want to rent or
purchase an automatic self-cycling electric pump. Even if you decide to
use a pump, you should still learn to hand express. Hand expression is
economical and easy, something every breastfeeding mother should know.

Your first tries at expressing milk may only produce enough milk to cover
the bottom of the collection container. Don't get discouraged. It may take

several days or weeks before you see an increase in the amount of milk obtained. Patience and practice are the keys to success. In the beginning you may want to express and collect from one breast while the baby breastfeeds from the opposite breast (Illustration 32). Infant suckling will stimulate a let-down reflex and increase the flow of milk. As your confidence grows, you may want to express milk early in the morning or between feedings when your breasts seem full. It is important that you establish a routine, relax, and think about your baby. This will encourage milk release and increase the amount of milk obtained.

HAND EXPRESSION

❧ Choose a quiet, comfortable place.

❧ Wash your hands with soap and water and rinse well.

❧ Put warm water on the breasts for 1–3 minutes. A warm shower or tub bath, warm washcloths, or soaking the breasts in a pan of warm water works well.

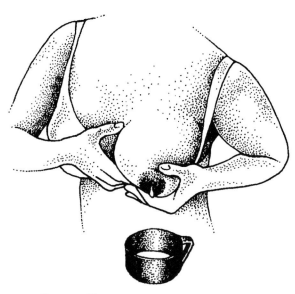

Illustration 33
Hand expression of breastmilk is economical and easy.
Patience and practice are the keys to success.

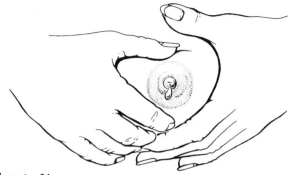

Illustration 34
During hand expression, change the position of your thumb and fingers on the breast until all parts of the breast are soft and the flow of milk slows down.

- Gently massage the breasts in a circular pattern using the flat part of your hand (Illustration 20).

- Roll your nipple between your thumb and finger. This will cause a let-down reflex and make milk expression easier.

- Relax and think about your baby. This will cause milk release and increase the amount of milk obtained.

- Gently support the breast with one or both hands.

- Place your thumb and first two fingers opposite each other just outside the edge of the areola, away from the nipple.

- Press in toward your chest, then slowly bring your thumb and fingers together, compressing the breast between your thumb and fingers. Do not squeeze or pinch. Do not compress the nipple itself (Illustration 33).

- Change the position of your thumb and fingers on the breast and repeat the press, compress motion until all parts of the breast have been expressed and the flow of milk slows down (5–10 minutes). Think of your breast as the face of a clock, and position your thumb and fingers at 6 and 12, 1 and 7, 2 and 8, and 3 and 9 (Illustration 34).

- Repeat the procedure on the opposite breast. You will need to express each breast several times, until the desired amount of milk has been collected or your breasts feel soft (20–30 minutes).

EXPRESSING WITH A BREAST PUMP

❧ Wash your hands with soap and water and rinse well.

❧ Put warm water on the breasts for 1–3 minutes. Warm washcloths, a warm shower or tub bath, or soaking the breasts in a pan of warm water works well.

❧ Gently massage the breasts in a circular pattern using the flat part of your hand.

❧ Roll your nipple between your thumb and finger. This will cause a let-down reflex and make milk expression easier.

❧ Relax and think about your baby. This will cause milk release and increase the amount of milk obtained.

❧ Adjust the suction control on the pump to the lowest setting. Moisten the pump horn (funnel) with water. Center your nipple in the opening. Follow the directions that come with each pump.

❧ Pump for 5–10 minutes or until the flow of milk slows down, rest 3–5 minutes, then repeat once or twice.

❧ Express each breast until the desired amount of milk has been obtained or the breasts feel soft. Refrigerate or freeze milk for later use. The collection container that comes with many pumps can be used for storage.

❧ Wash the pump after each use in hot, soapy water and rinse well. During work hours, rinse the pump in hot water and wash in hot, soapy water when you get home.

CHOOSING A BREAST PUMP

Some mothers rent or purchase a breast pump during the last weeks of pregnancy so they can get ready for their return to work. Once you hold your baby in your arms, you may find that plans made during pregnancy change. So you might want to wait until after your baby is born to choose a breast pump. The following suggestions will help you choose the pump that is right for you.

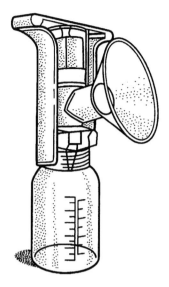

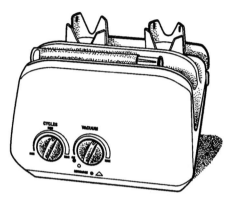

Illustration 35
Mothers who prefer to pump one breast
while the baby breastfeeds on the opposite
can use a squeeze-handle hand pump.
(Example shown is by Hollister®.)

Illustration 36
Mothers who plan to pump frequently
(1 or more times a day) should consider
an automatic self-cycling electric pump
that is much like a breastfeeding baby.
(Example shown is an Elite™ by Hollister®.)

Factors to consider include:

- reason for use
  (to increase your milk supply, to establish a milk supply, to provide
  an occasional supplement, to feed a preterm infant)
- frequency of use
- effectiveness
- ease of operation
- ease of cleaning
- availability
- durability
- cost

Features to look for include:

- pressure range
- suction control
- funnel size and shape
- storage capacity
- backflow protection

❧ Mothers who plan to pump now and then (once or twice a week) should consider hand expression, a hand pump, or a battery-operated pump.

❧ Mothers who prefer to pump one breast while the baby breastfeeds from the opposite breast should consider a squeeze-handle hand pump, a battery-operated pump, or a semi-automatic electric pump, all of which can be easily operated with one hand (Illustration 35).

❧ Mothers who plan to pump frequently (one or more times a day) should consider an automatic self-cycling electric pump (Illustration 36).

❧ An automatic self-cycling electric pump with a double collection kit that lets you pump both breasts at once saves time and energy (Illustration 24). In addition, double-pumping increases prolactin levels, which increases milk production.

Your first tries at pumping may only produce enough milk to cover the bottom of the collection container. Don't get discouraged. It may take several days or several weeks before you see an increase in the amount of milk obtained. Like breastfeeding, pumping is a learned art.

Your pumping method is equally as important as your choice of pump. Try to establish a routine.

❧ Choose a quiet, comfortable place.

❧ Put warm water on your breasts for 1–3 minutes.

❧ Gently massage your breast and roll your nipple between your thumb and finger to start the flow of milk.

❧ Relax and think about your baby. Looking at a picture of your baby, listening to music, or listening to a relaxation tape will increase the amount of milk obtained.[74]

❧ As with breastfeeding, patience and practice are the keys to success.

SUGGESTIONS FOR CHOOSING A BREAST PUMP

Reason for Use and/or Purchase	Hand Expression	Hand Pump	Battery Pump	Semi-Automatic Electric Pump	Self-Cycling Electric Pump
To begin a milk supply					☙
To increase a milk supply	☙	☙	☙	☙	☙
To provide an occasional supplement	☙	☙	☙	☙	
To provide human milk for a hospitalized preterm infant					☙
To pump 1–2 times a week	☙	☙	☙	☙	
To pump 1 or more times a day				☙	☙
To pump 1 breast while the baby breastfeeds from the opposite breast		☙	☙	☙	
To double pump				☙	☙

STORAGE OF HUMAN MILK

- For hand expression, use a container with a wide opening. A mayonnaise or peanut butter jar works best. Wash the container in hot, soapy water and rinse well or clean in a dishwasher.

- Pour the expressed milk into a plastic or glass container for storage. Allow room for expansion if you plan to freeze the milk.

- Label all containers with the time and date.

- Place a single serving in each container. More than one container can be thawed if larger amounts are needed. During the first 3 months, babies eat about 2½ oz. per lb. each day. For example, an 8 lb. baby would eat 2½ oz. x 8 lb. or 20 oz. per day. Divide the daily intake by the number of feedings and you can estimate

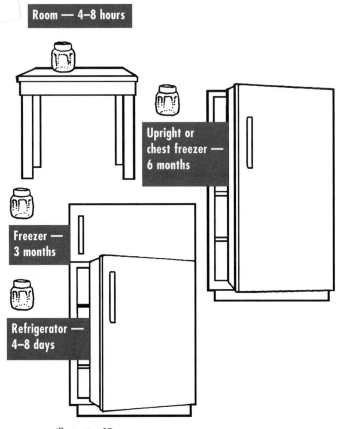

Illustration 37
Breastmilk storage recommendations for healthy babies.

the size of a single feeding. Since 20 oz. ÷10 feedings = 2 oz., the mother of an 8 lb. baby would want to freeze in 2 oz. servings.

🌱 Human milk for healthy, full term babies can be stored at room temperature for 4–8 hours, in the refrigerator for 4–8 days, in the freezer section of a refrigerator/freezer for 3 months, or in an upright or chest freezer for 6 months[74] (Illustration 37).

🌱 Human milk stored in the freezer should be placed in the middle of the freezer compartment. Do not store milk in the freezer door.

✦ To thaw, place the unopened container in the refrigerator or in a pan of warm water. Do not thaw in a microwave oven. A microwave oven destroys live cells and heats the milk unevenly, which increases the risk of burning the baby.[88]

✦ Serve breastmilk at room temperature. Heating destroys live cells and important nutrients.

✦ Human milk that has been thawed in the refrigerator should be used within 24 hours. Milk that has been thawed in a pan of warm water should be used within 4 hours. Any milk left in the feeding container (bottle, cup etc.) can be saved for the next feeding only.

✦ You can combine small amounts of breastmilk to make a single serving. If you combine fresh milk and frozen milk, chill the fresh milk in the refrigerator first to avoid thawing the frozen layer.

HUMAN MILK STORAGE RECOMMENDATIONS FOR HEALTHY, FULL TERM BABIES*

Human Milk	Room Temperature (25° C or 77° F)	Refrigerator (4° C or 39° F)	Refrigerator/Freezer (-5° C or 5° F)	Freezer (-20° C or -4° F)
Fresh	4–8 hours	4–8 days	3 months	6 months
Thawed in refrigerator	4 hours	24 hours	Do not refreeze	Do not refreeze
Thawed in pan of warm water	Use right away or refrigerate	4 hours	Do not refreeze	Do not refreeze

Fresh breastmilk is best for your baby. Storage recommendations may vary with your baby's age and health.

Weaning

Any amount of breastfeeding is good for you and your baby. How long you breastfeed depends on your own feelings and the needs of your baby. Mothers may choose to breastfeed for several weeks, several months, or several years. Some babies lose interest in breastfeeding between 6 and 12 months, when solid foods or a cup are introduced. Occasionally something happens that makes the separation of mother and baby, and weaning, necessary. More important than when you wean or why is that the process be slow. Weaning, particularly sudden weaning, may cause feelings of sadness and guilt. This is due to the sudden decrease in prolactin, as well as the unexpected end of the breastfeeding relationship. While these feelings are common and will pass with time, it may help to talk about them with people you trust.

SUGGESTIONS FOR WEANING SLOWLY

- Replace 1 breastfeeding at a time with solids or liquids, depending on the baby's age and ability. Choose a breastfeeding when the baby is least interested.

- Frequently babies refuse substitutes offered by mother. You might want to ask a brother, sister, or father to help with replacement feedings.

- Replace one breastfeeding every 3–5 days until weaning is complete.

- Increase cuddling time. Separation from the breast should not mean separation from mother.

- Distract an active and curious toddler with games, outdoor play, and story-telling.

- Offer foods that are not available from the breast, yet appeal to young children. Apple juice, grape juice, chocolate milk, and finger foods are suggested.

- Expect some milk production to continue for 4–6 weeks.

SUGGESTIONS FOR SUDDEN WEANING

- Hand express or pump a small amount of milk to relieve fullness and prevent engorgement. A warm washcloth, a warm shower or tub bath, or soaking the breasts in a pan of warm water may make milk expression easier. Remove only enough milk to relieve fullness. The more milk you remove, the more milk you will make.

- Put ice on the breasts to relieve pain and reduce swelling. Bags of frozen peas wrapped in wet washcloths work well.

- Wear a snug bra for comfort and support.

- Take acetaminophen or ibuprofen for pain.

Common Questions

Will breastfeeding change the size and shape of my breasts?
No. Breastfeeding does not change breast size and shape. Some women find that their breasts get smaller and sag or droop after birth. This is true whether you choose to breastfeed or bottle-feed. These changes are due to heredity, age, and weight gain. Usually, the more weight you gain during pregnancy, the more your breasts will shrink or sag when the added pounds are lost.

Can I breastfeed and still lose weight?
Yes. You need 500–1,000 calories each day for milk production in addition to the 1,800 calories your body needs. While you can add 500 calories to your diet and still lose weight, most mothers produce a good supply of milk while eating the same number of calories. Fat stored during pregnancy will usually satisfy your added calorie needs. Frequently mothers find that weight loss has never been easier and work instead to maintain their weight. However, if you are trying to lose unwanted pounds, avoid foods with little or no nutritional value.

Must I follow a special diet while breastfeeding?
No. As long as you eat a variety of foods (breads, fruits, vegetables, dairy products, proteins, and fats), and drink to satisfy your thirst, both you and your baby should be fine. Sometimes certain foods in a mother's diet make her baby fussy. Milk products, nuts, eggs, wheat, chocolate, and coffee or tea with caffeine may be the cause. Should this happen, you may need to limit that particular food.

Can I smoke while breastfeeding?
Yes and no. Cigarette smoking lowers the fat content of milk and decreases milk production. This may explain why mothers who smoke breastfeed for shorter periods of time. Smoking also increases the risk of Sudden Infant Death Syndrome (SIDS). Because the benefits of breastfeeding outweigh the risks of smoking, mothers who smoke are still encouraged to breastfeed. If possible, limit the number of cigarettes you smoke to fewer than 10 a day and do not smoke in the house or car or near the baby.[66, 67]

Can I drink alcohol while breastfeeding?

Yes and no. Alcohol passes easily into breastmilk. When a mother consumes 3 or 4 drinks a day, the alcohol can affect her baby's motor development (ability to crawl, walk, grasp, hold, etc.).[65] While small amounts of alcohol (1 or 2 drinks a day) are thought to be safe, even 1 or 2 drinks can affect a mother's ability to care for her baby. To reduce the effect of alcohol on you and your baby, drink no more than 1 or 2 drinks a week, and do not breastfeed for at least 2 hours after you drink.

Will certain foods change the color of my breastmilk?

Yes. Some mothers have reported orange, green, or black breastmilk when they eat certain foods or take certain medicines. If the color of your breastmilk changes from bluish white (foremilk) or creamy white (hindmilk) to another color, make a list of the foods or medicines you have taken that might be the cause. If the color change continues, call your doctor, your baby's doctor, or a lactation consultant. You can continue to breastfeed as long as your baby shows no signs of illness (vomiting, diarrhea, or fever).

Can I breastfeed if there is blood in my breastmilk?

Yes. Bleeding can occur if there is breast or nipple damage. Your breastmilk can be pink, red, or orange. If the cause of the bleeding is easily seen, you can put colostrum, breastmilk, or modified lanolin on the damaged area to aid healing. If the cause of the bleeding is not easily seen or if the bleeding lasts for several days, contact your doctor. While bleeding is seldom serious, bleeding can be a sign of breast cancer. You can continue to breastfeed as long as your baby shows no signs of illness (vomiting, diarrhea, or fever).

What if I become ill and need medicine?

Many medicines are safe for breastfeeding mothers and babies.[89] However, check with your doctor before taking any medicine, including those available without a prescription (over-the-counter). Remind your doctor that you are breastfeeding so that he or she can recommend a medicine that is safe yet effective.

Won't breastfeeding "tie me down"?

Yes and no. In the beginning, when babies are breastfeeding often, breastfeeding can be time-consuming. Once your milk supply is stable (about 6–12 weeks after birth), and your baby is breastfeeding less

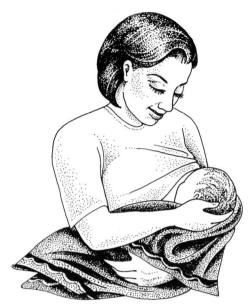

Illustration 38
With a little practice, mothers can breastfeed discreetly anywhere.

often, you will find it easier to come and go. If necessary, a substitute feeding can be given using expressed breastmilk or infant formula. You can use a cup, hollow-handled medicine spoon, medicine dropper, teaspoon, or bottle, whichever you prefer.

I want to breastfeed, but what if I find it embarrassing?

Some mothers feel embarrassed when they first start to breastfeed, others do not. How you will feel depends on your breastfeeding experience as well as the experience of those around you. Unfortunately, many people see the breast as a sexual object. As a result, many women are uncomfortable handling or exposing their breasts, even for something as natural and wonderful as breastfeeding. Be aware of your own feelings. If necessary, find a private place to breastfeed. Unplug the telephone. Put a small sign on your front door, "Hungry baby, do not disturb." With patience and practice your confidence in your choice to breastfeed will grow. Remember experienced mothers can breastfeed discreetly and modestly anywhere (Illustration 38).

How can I tell if my baby is getting enough to eat?
The amount of milk taken from the breasts at each feeding cannot be measured. As a result, many mothers worry about whether their babies are getting enough to eat. Remember one important fact about your baby, "Nothing comes out the bottom unless something goes in the top." The following signs will help to reassure you:

- Expect 3 stools a day for the first 3 days and at least 4 stools a day for the next 4 weeks.[39, 40]

  - Your baby's stool will be black and sticky (meconium) for several days. Once your baby is taking larger amounts of breastmilk, his stool will become watery and yellow, usually by the fourth day.

  - Breastfed babies' stools look like a mixture of water, yellow mustard, cottage cheese, and sesame seeds. Expect small, frequent, watery stools with very little solid material. Sometimes, a yellow stain the size of your baby's fist is all that you see.

- After the first 4–6 weeks, expect larger, softer, formed stools every 1–5 days.

- Expect at least 3 wet diapers a day during the first 3 days and at least 6 wet diapers a day after that. Disposable diapers absorb liquid so well that it is often hard to tell if a diaper is wet. To check for wetness, place several sheets of toilet paper inside the diaper when a new diaper is used.

- While wet diapers are important, a decrease in the number of stools is the first sign that your baby may not be getting enough to eat (see "Important Signs That Every Breastfeeding Parent Should Know," p. 145).

Do I need to give my baby vitamin and mineral supplements?
No. If you have a healthy, full-term baby, human milk provides all the vitamins (A, C, D, and E) and minerals (iron and fluoride) your baby needs for the first 6 months of life. Your baby will get a single dose of vitamin K after birth to prevent bleeding.[90] In addition, a daily dose of vitamin D is recommended for babies whose mothers are poorly nourished and for babies who are dark-skinned and get little sun exposure. Babies store enough iron in their liver during the last weeks of

pregnancy to meet their iron needs for 6 months. After 6 months, iron-fortified solid foods are recommended.

If I breastfeed, can I still give my baby a pacifier?
Yes and no. Pacifiers can confuse a baby's suckling pattern and decrease a mother's milk supply. Pacifiers also can increase the risk of ear infections and cause early weaning.[91, 92] During the early weeks, when you and your baby are learning to breastfeed, pacifiers should be avoided. After your baby is breastfeeding well (4–6 weeks after birth), and gaining weight (4–8 ounces a week), you can offer a pacifier. Many breast-fed babies choose to suck on their fists, thumbs, or fingers instead, and refuse pacifiers.

If my baby has colic can I still breastfeed?
Yes. Colic, long periods of fussing and crying each day for no clear reason, occurs in 10–20% of newborns. Colic occurs in formula-fed babies as well as breastfed babies. The symptoms usually appear 2–6 weeks after birth and disappear by 12–16 weeks of age. The cause of colic is unclear. Occasionally overfeeding or something in the infant's or the mother's diet can cause fussiness. Often no cause is found.

If you have a very fussy baby, offer 1 breast at each feeding.[16] The result will be a low volume, low sugar, high fat meal rather than a high volume, high sugar, low fat meal. In addition, avoid cow's milk-based formulas in your baby's diet and milk products, eggs, nuts, and wheat in your diet (see "Breastfeeding the Baby with a Family History of Allergic Disease," p. 106).

Constant sounds or vibrations like a vacuum cleaner, clothes dryer, car engine, or untuned television may soothe a fussy baby. A warm compress on the abdomen can also be helpful. A warm tub bath, a warm washcloth, or a warm water bottle works well. While colic seldom lasts more than 16 weeks, it can seem like 16 years! A mother unable to calm her baby feels guilty. A father unable to calm his partner feels helpless. If the fussiness continues, medicine can be helpful. You will need to call your baby's doctor for a prescription.

seldom necessary. Frequently, the use of infant formula symptoms worse. As the infant grows and the intestinal tract matures, the symptoms will improve. Remember, a normal infant cries 2–3 hours a day.[93]

I tried to breastfeed my first baby, but I was unable to produce enough milk. How can I keep this from happening again?
Almost every mother can produce enough milk to nourish her baby. Some women have a limited number of milk-producing cells (alveoli); however, this is rare.[94] When a mother's milk supply or a baby's weight gain is low, it is often the result of too little information, incorrect information, or too little support. The following suggestions will help you build and keep a good milk supply:

- Breastfeed whenever your baby seems fussy or hungry. During the early weeks, expect to breastfeed at least 8–12 times in 24 hours or every 1–3 hours during the day and every 2–3 hours at night. Sometimes a sleepy baby will not ask or demand to eat often enough. Therefore, during the first 4 weeks, keep your baby with you day and night. Watch for early signs of hunger or light sleep such as wiggling, lip smacking, finger sucking, yawning, or coughing, and offer the breast at those times.

- Breastfeed as long as the baby wishes on the first breast before offering the second breast. If the baby falls asleep while breastfeeding and the first breast is still firm and full, break the suction, burp him, wake him, and put him back on the first breast.

- Offer both breasts at every feeding. However, do not be concerned if your baby seems satisfied with one breast. Remember each breast can provide a full meal. It is more important that he breastfeed well on one breast than that he breastfeed on both breasts.

- Begin each feeding on the breast offered last.

- Avoid the use of water or formula supplements/substitutes during the first 4 weeks. Supplements/substitutes can confuse your baby's suckling pattern and limit breastmilk production.

❧ Drink to satisfy your thirst. Water and unsweetened fruit juices are suggested. It is not necessary to drink milk to make milk. Mothers who drink lots of milk or eat lots of milk products can have fussy babies.

❧ Eat a balanced diet.

❧ Get plenty of rest. Nap when the baby naps.

❧ Should problems occur, get help from people you trust.

How much weight should my baby gain in the beginning?
Your baby can lose up to 7% of his birth weight during the first week of life and should regain that weight during the second week. After the first or second week, your baby should gain 4–8 ounces a week. Sometimes a baby will gain less. However, breastfeeding patterns should be carefully reviewed.

Babies often double their birth weight by 4–6 months of age and triple their birth weight by 1 year of age.

I plan to give my baby a substitute feeding using expressed breastmilk. How much milk will I need to express for a feeding?
A healthy, full term baby needs about 2½ oz. per lb. each day (see "Estimate the Size of a Single Serving During the First 3 Months," p. 115). For example, an 8 lb. baby would require 2½ oz. x 8 lb. or 20 oz. a day. If the baby breastfeeds every 2–3 hours, or 10 times a day and eats 20 oz. a day, then he eats about 2 oz. at each feeding. To be on the safe side, express 3–4 oz. of breastmilk and store the milk in 2 oz. servings to avoid waste. You can use more than 1 serving if necessary.

Some mothers prefer to substitute with infant formula and choose a soy-based formula rather than a cow's milk-based formula. Ask your baby's doctor for a recommendation.

Will breastfeeding affect my sex life?
Some mothers have less desire for sex due to tiredness, fear of pregnancy, or fear of pain. Others find that breastfeeding alone provides enough touching and holding to satisfy their sexual needs. Still others are eager to have sex. Discuss your feelings openly with your partner.

Many breastfeeding mothers have dryness in the vagina (birth canal) that can cause pain during intercourse (sex). A water soluble lubricant such as K-Y Jelly may be helpful. Put a small amount around the opening of the vagina before having sex.

When you have sex, you may have a climax or orgasm. Orgasm causes the release of oxytocin from the brain. Oxytocin causes the release of milk from the breasts. Some fathers feel like they have to come to bed thirsty! To limit the leakage of milk from the breasts during sex, breast-feed your baby before making love.

If I breastfeed can I still get pregnant?
Yes and no. You can achieve natural child spacing with full or nearly full breastfeeding. However, if your breastfeeding schedule or routine limits the frequency or length of breastfeedings or includes frequent use of breastmilk substitutes, pregnancy is more likely.

Ovulation (egg release) and menstruation (monthly bleeding) may not occur while you are breastfeeding, especially during the first 6–12 weeks. However, most women resume ovulation and menstruation while breastfeeding. Ovulation can occur before menstruation; therefore, do not assume that you are protected (safe) until after your first menstrual period.

If pregnancy is not desired, a safe method of birth control is suggested. Your choices include cervical cap, female condom, diaphragm, intrauterine device, male condom, and spermicidal cream, foam, or jelly. Birth control pills that contain estrogen and progestin (combination pills) are not recommended (Illustration 1). However, birth control pills, implants (Norplant®), or injections (Depo-Provera®) that contain only progestin are safe (see "Common Concerns," p. 21). Discuss the choices with your doctor, midwife, lactation consultant, or nurse.

If I become pregnant can I still breastfeed?
Yes and no. Many mothers continue to breastfeed during pregnancy and have two babies or a baby and a child at the breast after birth. This is called tandem nursing. To meet the needs of two growing babies, you will need to eat a balanced diet that includes extra calories, drink to

satisfy your thirst, and nap when the babies nap. As long as the younger baby is fully breastfed and the older baby is taking some solid foods, you should breastfeed the younger baby first.

During pregnancy, a mother's breasts and nipples can become tender and the volume and content of her breastmilk changes. When breastmilk volume decreases, sodium and protein increase, and lactose and glucose (sugars) decrease, making the milk look and taste more like colostrum. Sometimes the older baby or child loses interest in the breast (child-led weaning) or the breast tenderness, common during pregnancy, makes breastfeeding painful, and weaning occurs (mother-led weaning).

Breastfeeding can cause uterine contractions but there is no evidence to suggest that the developing fetus (unborn baby) is at risk. However, if you have a history of premature labor or vaginal bleeding during pregnancy, your doctor or midwife may suggest that you wean (see "Weaning," p. 131).

Do I need to stop breastfeeding when the baby's teeth come in?
No. You do not need to wean when your baby's teeth come in. Both of my children got their first tooth at 3 months of age but were breastfed more than a year. Biting can occur at the end of a feeding, when the baby is no longer hungry, but playful. Simply remove the baby from the breast with a firm, "no." If the baby is still hungry, offer the breast again. If the biting continues, remove the baby from the breast for several minutes. Your baby will soon learn that biting brings an end to breastfeeding, and the biting will stop.

How long should I breastfeed?
Until you or your baby decide that it is time to stop. This may be several weeks, several months, or several years. Doctors recommend breastfeeding alone for the first 6 months. Then solid foods are slowly introduced, reducing the need for human milk. However, human milk or infant formula is necessary during the first year of life.[63] Many women choose to breastfeed until the baby can be weaned easily to solid foods and a cup (12–24 months). This avoids the added cost of bottles and formula.

What are growth spurts?

Growth spurts or frequency days often occur around 3 weeks, 6 weeks, 3 months, and 6 months. However, growth spurts can occur at any time. Your baby may be fussy and restless and want to breastfeed all the time. Well-meaning but inexperienced friends and relatives may suggest that "your milk isn't rich enough," that "you're not making enough milk," that "solid foods or formula supplements are necessary," or that "it is time to stop breastfeeding." After 2–3 days of frequent breastfeedings, your milk supply will catch up with the increased demand, and the length and frequency of breastfeedings will decrease. Feeling confident in your ability to breastfeed your baby is very important. Seek advice from experienced friends or relatives or a certified lactation consultant (IBCLC) in your community.

What are nursing strikes?

A nursing strike occurs when a baby suddenly refuses to breastfeed. It can last for several feedings or several days. Sometimes the cause is easily identified, such as teething, fever, ear infection, stuffy nose (cold), constipation, or diarrhea. Occasionally, menstruation (monthly bleeding) or something in your diet will change the taste of your milk. Deodorant, perfume, or powder placed on the mother's skin can be the cause of the strike. Frequently no cause is found. Until the strike ends, you will need to hand express or pump to relieve fullness and maintain your milk supply. Continue to offer the breast. However, do not insist if the baby refuses. Give expressed breastmilk by teaspoon, eye dropper, hollow-handled medicine spoon, or cup until breastfeeding resumes. Be patient and relax. Watch for early signs of hunger and offer the breast at those times. Limit noise and distractions during feedings. Give your baby undivided attention. Nursing strikes seldom lead to weaning. With time, the baby will return to the breast.

Can I breastfeed if I am HIV positive?

The Centers for Disease Control and Prevention (CDC) and the World Health Organization (WHO) recommend that HIV positive women not breastfeed, as long as they live in countries where there are clean, safe supplies (water, formula, bottles, and nipples) available to feed their babies. However, in countries where the risk of death during the first year of life from diarrhea and other infections is high (greater than 50%), breastfeeding is encouraged, even among HIV positive women.

Can I breastfeed if I use illegal drugs?
Women who are chemically dependent and actively abusing drugs should not breastfeed. However, recovering drug users who remain drug-free can breastfeed. Close follow-up is recommended for both the mother and the baby.[95]

Can I exercise if I am breastfeeding?
Yes. Moderate exercise does not affect the amount of milk produced. However, exercise can increase the level of lactic acid in the milk and give the milk a sour taste. In addition, some babies dislike the taste of the sweat on the mother's skin and refuse to breastfeed. If this occurs, rinse the breasts before you breastfeed or breastfeed no sooner than 1½ hours after exercising.[96, 97]

I had breast surgery. Will I be able to breastfeed?
Yes and no. Breast surgery can affect your ability to produce milk. However, many women who have had breast surgery breastfeed fully (without water, juice, or formula supplements). Talk with your doctor about your concerns.

The most common surgical procedures are breast augmentation (insertion of implants), breast reduction (removal of breast tissue), lumpectomy (removal of a breast lump), and masectomy (removal of a breast). Your ability to breastfeed will depend upon the location of the incision and the extent of the surgery, If the incision is near the nipple and areola, damage to milk ducts, nerves, and blood vessels is more likely. Women who have had a masectomy can breastfeed fully on the remaining breast, but may need to breastfeed more often in the beginning to increase their milk supply.

Women who have had breast reduction surgery often find that milk production is limited.[98] When a large amount of breast tissue is removed, nipples are frequently repositioned on the newly formed breasts, damaging milk ducts, nerves, and blood vessels. While women who have had breast reduction surgery are encouraged to breastfeed, they need to know that supplementation may be necessary if their babies gain less than 4–8 ounces a week. Remember to tell your baby's doctor that you have had breast surgery and be sure to check your baby's weight often (once a week) during the early weeks.

Can I breastfeed if I have silicone breast implants?
Yes. Women with silicone breast implants, as well as other implants, can breastfeed, as long as the implants are not leaking.[99] Talk with your doctor about your concerns.

When should I call my baby's doctor?
Problems can occur during the early weeks when a mother and baby are learning to breastfeed. You can prevent serious problems if you know the early warning signs that your baby may not be getting enough to eat. If your baby is less than 6 weeks of age and **any** of the following occur, **call your baby's doctor:**

- fewer than 3 bowel movements a day during the first 3 days or fewer than 4 bowel movements a day during the next 4 weeks

- fewer than 3 wet diapers a day during the first 3 days or fewer than 6 wet diapers a day during the next 4 weeks

- fewer than 8 breastfeedings a day

- no sign of suckling and swallowing (milk transfer) when breastfeeding

- no sign of milk release (let-down)

- your baby is either restless and fussy or listless and sleepy for long periods of time

- your baby has lost more than 7% of his birth weight

- your baby is below birth weight at 2 weeks of age

- your baby is gaining less than 4–8 oz. a week

IMPORTANT SIGNS THAT EVERY BREASTFEEDING PARENT SHOULD KNOW

SIGNS THAT YOUR BABY IS WELL FED	SIGNS THAT YOUR BABY MAY NOT BE GETTING ENOUGH TO EAT
Your baby is alert and active.	Your baby is sleepy and listless.
Your baby is content after breastfeeding.	Your baby is restless and fussy after breastfeeding.
Your baby breastfeeds at least 8 times in 24 hours.	Your baby breastfeeds fewer than 8 times in 24 hours.
You can hear or see your baby swallow when he breastfeeds.	There is no sign of swallowing when your baby breastfeeds.
Your baby loses less than 7% of his birth weight during the first week.	Your baby loses more than 7% of his birth weight during the first week.
Your baby is back to his birth weight by 2 weeks of age.	Your baby is below his birth weight at 2 weeks of age.
Your baby is gaining 4–8 oz. a week.	Your baby is gaining less than 4 oz. a week.
Your baby is having at least 4 stools and 6 wet diapers a day by the fourth day.	Your baby is having fewer than 4 stools and 6 wet diapers a day by the fourth day.

© *Amy Spangler's Breastfeeding, A Parent's Guide. All rights reserved.*

Conclusion

Breastfeeding is a wonderful part of parenting — a chance to hold, to touch, to know your baby from the first moment of birth. Human milk is nature's way of protecting and nourishing your baby.

During the early 1900s efforts were made to improve upon nature. A tremendous amount of time and money was spent developing breastmilk substitutes. Infant feeding became a science of mixing and measuring. Mothers, fathers, and babies were separated at birth. Rules and routines were strictly enforced. Breastfeeding became the exception, while bottle-feeding became the norm. Parents choosing to breastfeed and professionals choosing to recommend breastfeeding had to justify the use of human milk for human infants. Routine use of breastmilk substitutes became the largest uncontrolled experiment in medical history. As a result, there was a significant increase in infant infection and infant death.[100] The advantages of breastfeeding as well as the dangers of bottle-feeding were quite clear.

Today the World Health Organization, the United States Department of Health and Human Services, and the American Academy of Pediatrics are working together to promote breastfeeding worldwide.[101, 102] Every effort is being made to identify the barriers that keep parents from beginning to breastfeed or continuing to breastfeed.[103] Too little information, incorrect information, too little support, and early use of breastmilk substitutes are just a few examples. Barriers exist in the hospital as well as the workplace. Hospital routines and inflexible work schedules that separate mothers and babies and limit the length and frequency of breastfeedings make it difficult for mothers to continue breastfeeding.

Most parents today know that breastfeeding is the best choice for every baby. Now parents need to know that breastfeeding is the right choice for every parent as well, that breastfeeding can be flexible, that breastfeeding can be fun.

Enjoyment is the measure of success. A firm desire to breastfeed, a clear understanding of how to proceed, and encouragement and support from people you trust will increase your enjoyment of breastfeeding and assure your success. While breastfeeding is the natural way to feed your baby, breastfeeding does not always come naturally. It is a learned skill that requires preparation, practice, and encouragement. Your partner, grand-mother, mother, sister, friend, doctor, nurse, lactation consultant, and childbirth educator are good sources of support. So don't hesitate to ask for help. With practice and patience your confidence in your ability to breastfeed will grow.

Regardless of your feeding choice, parenting is a tremendous challenge. It is the most difficult job you will ever do with the least amount of preparation. You will work 24 hours a day, 7 days a week, 52 weeks a year. Your salary will be a smile, a laugh, a hug, a first word, a first step, a first tooth — and without hesitation, you would do it all again. Parenting is a special joy. Cherish each moment.

While breastfeeding may not seem the right choice for every parent, it is the best choice for every baby.

References

1. National Academy of Science: *Nutrition During Lactation*. Washington, DC: National Academy Press, 1991.

2. Dewey KG et al: Maternal weight-loss patterns during prolonged lactation. *Am J Clin Nutr* 58: 162–66, 1993.

3. Butte NF et al: Effect of maternal diet and body composition on lactational performance. *Am J Clin Nutr* 39: 296–306, 1984.

4. Michels KB et al: Prospective assessment of breastfeeding and breast cancer incidence among 89,887 women. *Lancet* 347: 431–436, 1996.

5. Newcomb PA et al: Lactation and a reduced risk of premenopausal breast cancer. *New England Journal of Medicine* 330(2): 82–87, 1993.

6. Rosenblatt KA et al: Prolonged lactation and endometrial cancer. *Int J Epidemiology* 24(3): 499–503, 1995.

7. Rosenblatt KA et al: Lactation and the risk of epithelial ovarian cancer. *Int J Epidemiology* 22(2): 192–197, 1993.

8. Kalkwarf HJ et al: Intestinal calcium absorption of women during lactation and after weaning. *Am J Clin Nutr* 63: 526–531,1996.

9. Labbock M et al: The Lactational Amenorrhea Method (LAM): A postpartum introductory family planning method with policy and program implications. *Advances in Contraception* 10(2): 93–109, 1994.

10. Montgomery, DL et al: Economic benefit of breastfeeding infants enrolled in WIC. *Journal American Dietetic Association* 97(4): 379–385, 1997.

11. Dewey KG, Nommsen-Rivers LA: Differences in morbidity between breast-fed and formula-fed infants. *Journal of Pediatrics* 126: 696–702, 1995.

12. Scariati PD et al: A longitudinal analysis of infant morbidity and the extent of breastfeeding in the United States. *Pediatrics* 99(6): e5, 1997.

13. Wright AL et al: Increasing breastfeeding rates to reduce infant illness at the community level. *Pediatrics* 101: 837–844, 1998.

14. Cohen R et al: Comparison of maternal absenteeism and infant illness rates among breastfeeding and formula-feeding women in two corporations. *American Journal of Health Promotion* 10(2): 148–153, 1995.

15. Wagner CL et al: Special properties of human milk. *Clinical Pediatrics* June: 283–293, 1996.

16. Woolridge MW et al: Colic, "overfeeding," and symptoms of lactose malabsorption in the breastfed baby: A possible artifact of feed management? *Lancet* August: 382–384, 1988.

17. Pickering LK et al: Modulation of the immune system by human milk and infant formula containing nucleotides. *Pediatrics* 101(2): 242–249, 1998.

18. Bardare M et al: Influence of dietary manipulation on incidence of atopic disease in infants at risk. *Annals of Allergy* 71: 366–371, 1993.

19. Bruno G et al: Prevention of atopic diseases in high risk babies (long term follow-up). *Allergy Practice* 14: 181–187, 1993.

20. Saarinen UM et al: Breastfeeding as prophylaxsis against atopic disease: Prospective follow-up study until 17 years old. *Lancet* 346: 1065–1069, 1995.

21. Popkins BM et al: Breastfeeding and diarrheal morbidity. *Pediatrics* 86(6): 874–882, 1990.

22. Piscane A et al: Breastfeeding and urinary tract infection. *Journal of Pediatrics* 120(1): 87–89, 1992.

23. Beaudry M et al: Relation between infant feeding and infections during the first six months of life. *Journal of Pediatrics* 126: 191–197, 1995.

24. Duncan B et al: Exclusive breast-feeding for at least 4 months protects against otitis media. *Pediatrics* 91(5): 867–872, 1993.

25. Greco L et al: Case control study on nutritional risk factors in celiac disease. *Journal of Pediatric Gastroenterol Nutr* 7: 395–399, 1988.

26. Koletzko S et al: Role of infant feeding practices in development of Crohn's disease in childhood. *British Medical Journal* 298: 1617–1618, 1989.

27. Rigas et al: Breastfeeding and maternal smoking in the etiology of Crohn's disease and ulcerative colitis in childhood. *Ann Epidemiology* 3: 387–392, 1993.

28. Mayer EJ et al: Reduced risk of IDDM among breastfed children. *Diabetes* 37: 1625–1632, 1988.

29. Virtanen SM et al: Infant feeding in Finnish children <7 Yr of age with newly diagnosed IDDM. *Diabetes Care* 14: 415–417, 1991.

30. Shu X-O et al: Infant Breastfeeding and the risk of childhood lymphoma and leukaemia. *International Journal of Epidemiology* 24: 27–32, 1995.

31. Horwood LJ, Fergusson DM: Breastfeeding and later cognitive and academic outcomes. *Pediatrics* 101(1), 1998.

32. Lucas A et al: Breastmilk and subsequent intelligence quotient in children born preterm. *Lancet* 339: 261–264, 1992.

33. Fleming PJ et al: Environment of infants during sleep and risk of the sudden infant death syndrome: results of 1993–5 case-control study for confidential inquiry into stillbirths and deaths in infancy. *British Medical Journal* 313: 191–195, 1996.

34. Ford RPK et al: Breastfeeding and the risk of sudden infant death syndrome. *International Journal of Epidemiology* 22(5): 885–890, 1993.

35. Mitchell EA et al: Four modifiable and other major risk factors for cot death: The New Zealand study. *Journal of Paediatric Child Health* 28 (Suppl 1): S3–8, 1992.

36. McKenna JJ et al: Bedsharing promotes breastfeeding. *Pediatrics* 100(2): 214–219, 1997.

37. Mosko S et al: Infant arousals during mother-infant bed sharing: Implications for infant sleep and sudden infant death syndrome research. *Pediatrics* 100(5): 841–848, 1997.

38. Zeimer MM et al: Skin changes and pain in the nipple during the 1st week of lactation. *JOGNN* 22(3): 247–256, 1993.

39. Nyhan WL: Stool frequency of normal infants in the first week of life. *Pediatrics* 10(4): 414–425, 1952.

40. Shrago, L: Neonatal bowel output study (unpublished): AWHONN Conference (Research presentation) June 1996.

41. Pinilla T, Birch LL: Help me make it through the night: Behavioral entrainment of breast-fed infants' sleep patterns. *Pediatrics* 91(2): 436–443, 1993.

42. Hatcher RA et al: *Contraceptive Technology,* 17th edition. New York: Ardent Media, Inc., pp. 592–595, 1998.

43. Hatcher RA et al: *Contraceptive Technology,* 17th edition. New York: Ardent Media, Inc., pp. 602–604, 1998.

44. Kennedy KI et al: Premature introduction of progestin-only contraceptive methods during lactation. *Contraception* 55: 347–350, 1997.

45. Wright A et al: Changing hospital practices to increase the duration of breastfeeding. *Pediatrics* 97(5): 669–675, 1996.

46. Righard L et al: Effect of delivery room routines on success of first breastfeed. *Lancet* 36: 1105–1107, 1990.

47. Yamauchi Y et al: Breastfeeding frequency during the first 24 hours after birth in full-term neonates. *Pediatrics* 86(2): 171–175, 1990.

48. Nylander G et al: Unsupplemented breastfeeding in the maternity ward. Positive long-term effects. *Acta Obstetricia et Gynecologica Scandinavica* 70(3): 205–209, 1991.

49. Woolridge MW: The "anatomy" of infant sucking. *Midwifery* 2: 164–171, 1986.

50. Frantz KB: Managing nipple problems. *Exerpta Medica* 319–321, 1980.

51. Wiessinger, D: A breastfeeding teaching tool using a sandwich analogy for latch-on. *Journal of Human Lactation* 14(1): 51–56, 1998.

52. Righard L et al: Breastfeeding pattern: comparing the effects of infant behavior and maternal satisfaction of using one or two breasts. *Birth* 20(4): 182–185, 1993.

53. Woolridge MW et al: Do changes in pattern of breast usage alter the baby's nutrient intake? *Lancet* August: 395–397, 1990.

54. Humenick SS: The clinical significance of breastmilk maturation rates. *Birth* 14(4): 174–181, 1987.

55. Lawrence RA: *Breastfeeding a guide for the medical profession*, 5th edition. St. Louis: C.V. Mosby Company, pp. 248–249, 1999.

56. Alexander JM et al: Randomised controlled trial of breast shells and Hoffman's exercises for inverted and non-protractile nipples. *BMJ* 304: 1030–1032, 1992.

57. Auerbach KG: The effect of nipple shields on maternal milk volume. *JOGNN* 19(5): 419–427, 1990.

58. Hewat RJ, Ellis DJ: A comparison of the effectiveness of two methods of nipple care. *Birth* 14: 41, 1987.

59. Newton N: Nipple pain and nipple damage, Problems in the management of breastfeeding. *Journal of Pediatrics* 41: 411–423, 1952.

60. Righard L et al: Sucking technique and its effect on success of breastfeeding. *Birth* 19: 185–189, 1992.

61. Spangler AK, Hildebrandt E: The effect of modified lanolin on nipple pain/damage during the first ten days of breastfeeding. *IJCE* 8(3): 15–19, 1993.

62. Yamauchi Y et al: The relationship between rooming-in/not rooming-in and breastfeeding variables. *Acta Paediatr Scand* 79: 1017–1022, 1990.

63. Academy of Pediatrics Work Group on Breastfeeding: Breastfeeding and the Use of Human Milk. *Pediatrics* 100(6): 1035–1039, 1997.

64. Chandra RK: Five-year follow-up of high-risk infants with a family history of allergy who were exclusively breastfed or fed partial whey hydrolysate, soy, and conventional cow's milk formulas. *Journal of Pediatric Gastroenterology and Nutrition* 24(4): 380–388, 1997.

65. Little RE et al: Maternal alcohol use during breastfeeding and infant mental and motor development at one year. *New England Journal of Medicine* 321(7): 425–430, 1989.

66. Hopkinson, JM et al: Milk production by mothers of premature infants: Influence of cigarette smoking. *Pediatrics* 90(6): 934–938, 1992.

67. Horta BL et al: Environmental tobacco smoke and breastfeeding. *American Journal of Epidemiology* 146(2): 128–133, 1997.

68. Nikodem VC et al: Do cabbage leaves prevent breast engorgement? A randomized, controlled study. *Birth* 20: 61, 1993.

69. Roberts KL et al: Effects of cabbage leaf extract on breast engorgement. *Journal of Human Lactation* 14(3): 231–236, 1998.

70. Mathur et al: Anti-infective factors in preterm human colostrum. *Acta Paediatr Scand* 79: 1039–1044, 1990.

71. Lucas A, Cole TJ: Breastmilk and neonatal necrotising enterocolitis. *Lancet* 336: 1519, 1990.

72. Lucas A et al: Breastmilk and subsequent intelligence quotient in children born preterm, *Lancet* 339: 261–264, 1992.

73. Feher S et al: Increasing breastmilk production for premature infants with a relaxation/imagery audiotape. *Pediatrics* 83(1): 57, 1989.

74. Hamosh M et al: Breastfeeding and the working mother: Effect of time and temperature of short-term storage on proteolysis, lipolysis, and bacterial growth in milk. *Pediatrics* 97(4): 492, 1996.

75. Pardou A et al: Human Milk Banking: Influence of Storage Processes and of Bacterial Contamination on Some Milk Constituents. *Biol Neonate* 65:302-309, 1994.

76. Charpak N et al: Kangaroo mother versus traditional care for newborn infants <2000 grams: A randomized, controlled trial. *Pediatrics* 100: 682–688, 1997.

77. Meier P, Anderson GC: Responses of small preterm infants to bottle- and breastfeeding. *MCN* 12: 97, 1987.

78. Stutte PC et al: The effects of breast massage on volume and fat content of human milk. *Genesis* 10(2): 22, 1988.

79. Neifert M et al: Nipple confusion: Toward a formal definition. *Journal of Pediatrics* 26: S125–129, 1995.

80. Ehrenkranz RA et al: Metoclopramide effect on faltering milk production by mothers of premature infants. *Pediatrics* 78(4): 614, 1986.

81. Widstrom AM et al: Gastric suction in healthy newborn infants. *Acta Paediatr Scand* 76: 566–572, 1987.

82. Zinaman MJ et al: Acute prolactin and oxytocin responses and milk yield to infant suckling and artificial methods of expression in lactating women. *Pediatrics* 89(3): 437–440, 1992.

83. Gartner, LM: Neonatal jaundice. *Pediatrics in Review* 15(11): 422–432, 1994.

84. Brown LP et al: Incidence and pattern of jaundice in healthy breastfed infants during the first month of life. *Nursing Research* 42(2): 106–110, 1993.

85. Martinez JC et al: Hyperbilirubinemia in the breastfed newborn: A controlled trial of four interventions, *Pediatrics* 91(2): 470, 1993.

86. Zeiger RS: Development and prevention of allergic disease in childhood, *Allergy Principles and Practice*, 4th edition. St. Louis: C.V. Mosby Company, Vol II: pp. 1137–1167, 1993.

87. Ashad SH et al: The effect of genetic and environmental factors on the prevalence of allergic disorders at the age of two years. *Clinical Experimental Allergy* 23: 504–511, 1993.

88. Quan R et al: Effects of microwave radiation on anti-infective factors in human milk. *Pediatrics* 89: 667, 1992.

89. Hale TW: *Medications and Mother's Milk*, 6th edition. Amarillo, Texas: Pharmasoft Publishing, 1998.

90. Greer FR et al: Vitamin K status of lactating mothers, human milk, and breastfeeding infants. *Pediatrics* 88(4): 751–756, 1991.

91. Barros FC et al: Use of pacifiers is associated with decreased breastfeeding duration. *Pediatrics* 95(4): 497, 1995.

92. Victora CG et al: Pacifier use and short breastfeeding duration: Cause, consequence or coincidence? *Pediatrics* 99(3): 445–453, 1997.

93. St. James-Roberts I: Persistent infant crying. *Arch Diseases Childhood* 66: 653, 1991.

94. Neifert MR et al: Lactation failure due to insufficient glandular development of the breast. *Pediatrics* 76(5): 823–827, 1985.

95. Wilton J: Breastfeeding and the Chemically Dependent Woman, *NAACOG'S Clinical Issues in Perinatal and Women's Health Nursing* 3(4): 667, 1992.

96. Dewey KG et al: A randomized study of the effects of aerobic exercise by lactating women on breast-milk volume and composition. *New Eng J Med* 330(7): 449–453, 1994.

97. Wallace JP et al: Infant acceptance of postexercise breastmilk. *Pediatrics* 89(6): 1245, 1992.

98. Hurst NM: Lactation after augmentation mammoplasty. *Obstetrics & Gynecology* 87: 30–34, 1996.

99. Kjoller K et al: Health outcomes in offspring of mothers with breast implants. *Pediatrics* 102: 1112–1115, 1998.

100. Cunningham AS: Breastfeeding and health in the 1980s: A global epidemiologic review. *Journal of Pediatrics* 118(5): 659–666, 1991.

101. *Report of the Surgeon General's workshop on breastfeeding and human lactation.* Publication no. HRS-D-MC 84-2, U.S. Department of Health and Human Services, 1984.

102. *Followup report: The Surgeon General's workshop on breastfeeding and human lactation.* Publication no. HRS-D-MC 85-2, U.S. Department of Health and Human Services, 1985.

103. Spisak S, Gross SS: *Second followup report: The Surgeon General's workshop on breastfeeding and human lactation.* Washington, D.C.: National Center for Education in Maternal and Child Health, 1991.

Resources

To find an International Board Certified Lactation Consultant (IBCLC)* in your area contact:

International Lactation Consultant Association
4101 Lake Boone Trail, Suite 201
Raleigh, NC 27607-6518
Telephone: 919.787.5181
Facsimile: 919.787.4916
E-mail: ilca@erols.com
Website: www.ilca.org

*An International Board Certified Lactation Consultant (IBCLC) is a health care professional with special skills in lactation and breastfeeding management. To become an IBCLC, an individual must pass an independent examination administered by the International Board of Lactation Consultant Examiners (IBLCE).

To find a LaLeche League Leader* in your area contact:

LaLeche League International
1400 North Meacham Road
Schaumburg, IL 60168-4079
Telephone: 800.525.3243
Facsimile: 847.519.0035
E-mail: LLLHQ@llli.org
Website: www.lalecheleague.org

*A LaLeche League Leader is an experienced mother who has breastfed her own children and who has been trained by LaLeche League International to answer your questions.

Index

About the Author

Amy Spangler is a mother, nurse, author, lecturer, and recognized authority on the subject of breastfeeding. She holds a bachelor's degree in nursing from the Ohio State University and a master's degree in maternal and infant health from the University of Florida.

Amy has been teaching parent education classes for 30 years. Currently, she is Parent Education Coordinator for a private Ob/Gyn facility where she teaches breastfeeding, prenatal nutrition, prenatal exercise, preparation for labor and birth, infant CPR, and early pregnancy classes. She has worked as a labor and delivery nurse, office nurse, surgical assistant, and clinical instructor in a college of nursing.

A registered nurse and an international board certified lactation consultant, Amy is a former president of the International Lactation Consultant Association and a member of the International Childbirth Education Association, the Association of Women's Health, Obstetric, and Neonatal Nurses, and La Leche League International.

She lives in Atlanta, Georgia with her husband Dennis, a private practice physician, and their two sons, Matthew and Adam.

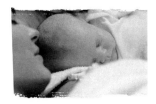

Additional copies of this book may be ordered by contacting:
Amy Spangler/Daddy, Mommy, and Me
P.O. Box 501046
Atlanta, Georgia 31150-1046

Telephone: 770.913.9332
Fax: 770.913.0822
E-mail: akspangler@daddymommyandme.com